PLAYING WITH

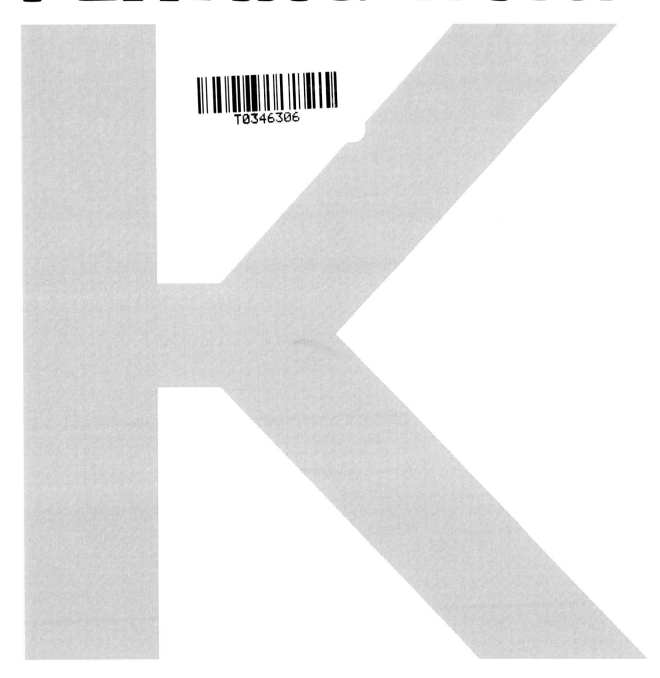

T0346306

Lucy Sanctuary

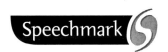

Published by

Speechmark Publishing Ltd, Sunningdale House, 43 Caldecotte Lake Drive,
Milton Keynes MK7 8LF, United Kingdom
Tel: +44 (0)1908 277177   Fax: +44 (0)1908 278297
www.speechmark.net

Copyright © Lucy Sanctuary, 2013

Designed by Moo Creative (Luton)

All rights reserved. The whole of this work, including all text and illustrations, is protected by copyright. No part of it may
be copied, altered, adapted or otherwise exploited in any way without express prior permission, unless in accordance with
the provisions of the Copyright Designs and Patents Act 1988 or in order to photocopy or make duplicating masters of
those pages so indicated, without alteration and including copyright notices, for the express purpose of instruction and
examination. No parts of this work may otherwise be loaded, stored, manipulated, reproduced, or transmitted in any form
or by any means, electronic or mechanical, including photocopying and recording, or by any information storage and
retrieval system without prior written permission from the publisher, on behalf of the copyright owner.

002-5799 - Printed in the United Kingdom by CMP (uk) Ltd

British Library Cataloguing in Publication Data
A catalogue record for this book is available from the British Library.

ISBN: 978 0 86388 923 3

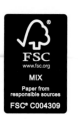

CONTENTS

ACKNOWLEDGEMENTS

I would like to thank:

Jo Gilmore for her support and advice, for being an amazing speech and language therapist and an even more amazing friend;

Sarah Norman and Judy Avery, for their encouragement and support;

Frances and Claire Burnham, Una Kroll and Tracey Fricker for putting up with me throughout the writing of this book;

Hilary and Stephanie for giving me this opportunity;

all the children who have played these games and enabled me to write this book.

This book is dedicated to my lovely children, Phoebe and Felix Sanctuary.

Many thanks to my mother, Maureen Baylis, for her endless support.

INTRODUCTION

Why do some children need support to use speech sounds?

Children usually start saying single words by 12 months (Flynn & Lancaster, 1996). By four and a half years, most children can use nearly all of the 24 consonant speech sounds that are in the English language, for example **m**, **b**, **p**, **s**, **k**. These speech sounds follow a developmental order: most children start saying the speech sounds **m**, **n**, **b**, **p**, **t**, **d**, **w** between 18 months and two years of age (Grunwell, 1985).

The development of speech sounds in children's talking. *(Source: Grunwell, 1985)*

One and a half years old to two years old	m, n, p, b, t, d, w
Two years old to two and a half years old	m, n, p, b, t, d, w Some children start saying **h**, **k**, **g** and **ng** (as in ing). These sounds are made at the back of the mouth.
Two and a half to three years old	m, n, p, b, t, d, w, h, k, g, ng, f, s, y Some children start to say **l**.
Three years to three and a half years old	m, n, p, b, t, d, w, h, k, g, ng, f, s, y, l Some children start to say **ch** and **sh**.
Three and a half to four and a half years old	m, n, p, b, t, d, w, h, k, g, ng, f, s, z, y, l (yes thanks!) **sh**, **ch**, **j** Some children start to say **r**.

However, not all children acquire the consonant speech sounds in the typical developmental order. For example, some children need help to say **k** and **g**, which are speech sounds made at the back of the mouth. They often use the earlier-developing speech sounds **t** and **d**, which are made at the front of the mouth, instead of **k** and **g**, in their talking.

There are various reasons why some children need support to use speech sounds. Listed below are some factors that can affect the development of speech sounds.

- Hearing impairments.
- Some children have frequent colds and ear infections such as glue ear, which can make it difficult for them to hear speech sounds accurately. We need to be

able to hear a speech sound clearly in order to copy it and say it accurately. Difficulties hearing a speech sound can result in difficulties saying it.

- Attention and listening difficulties and short concentration spans can result in difficulties hearing speech sounds accurately. Children with these difficulties often miss important visual information about how we say speech sounds, for example the shape of our lips, where we put the tongue. This can affect the child's ability to say speech sounds correctly.

- Some children develop more slowly than others and need more time to use speech sounds (developmental delay).

- Children need to hear people talking in order to learn how to use speech sounds. Lack of opportunities to hear speech can affect the development of speech sounds.

- Using a dummy or sucking a bottle until two and a half or three can restrict the range of tongue movements a child makes, and this can affect their speech. For example, some children who use a dummy for a long time say the speech sounds **k** and **g**, which are made at the back of the mouth, instead of the speech sounds **t** and **d**, which are made at the front of the mouth. This is because the dummy restricts movement of the tongue tip, which we use to say the speech sounds **t** and **d**.

- Some children have difficulty coordinating the movements needed for speech, for example tongue movements, lip movements, breath support, because they have speech disorders or developmental verbal dyspraxia (DVD). Developmental verbal dyspraxia 'is a condition where the child has difficulty in making and co-ordinating the precise movements which are used in the production of spoken language, although there is no damage to muscles or nerves' (Ripley *et al,* 1997). The child knows what they want to tell you, but difficulties co-ordinating the precise movements needed to say it (for example sequencing tongue movements and lip movements), can make it very hard for listeners to understand. In other words, what the child says does not match what they want to say: 'My mouth won't co-operate with my brain' (quote from Kevin, aged 13, in Stackhouse, 1992).

- Speech sound difficulties are often found in families, so there might be other family members who have had help to say speech sounds accurately.

How does difficulty using speech sounds affect children?

Children with speech sound difficulties are often hard for people outside the family to understand. Children can become reluctant to talk as they are worried that others will not understand what they want to say. Speech sound difficulties can prevent a child from taking part in nursery and classroom activities and limit their ability to express themselves – to ask questions, to give opinions, to tell stories, etc. Children often worry that, if they put up their hand to answer a question, no one will understand what they say and other children might laugh at them. Communication difficulties can lead to low self-confidence and low self-esteem.

The speech sound k

You may like to know that:

- Most children start to say the speech sound **k** at around two and a half to three years of age (Grunwell, 1985).

- We make the speech sound **k** at the back of our mouths, by lifting the back of the tongue to touch the top of the mouth. Say **cow** and feel the back of the tongue lift and block the air from coming out of the mouth. When the tongue lowers, the air is released in a little explosion and you say **k**. If you put your hand in front of your mouth when you say **cow** you can feel the air released. This can help children to say **k**. Using a mirror to show the child how to say **k**, for example by lifting the back of the tongue, can help them say the speech sound.

- The speech sound **k** is a quiet sound, not a noisy speech sound like **g**.

- The speech sound **k** is a short sound, not a long speech sound like **s**.

- The speech sound **k** is not the same as the letter (grapheme) **k**. When we say the letter **k**, we say **kay**.

- The letter **c** sometimes sounds like the speech sound **k**, e.g. **cat**, and sometimes sounds like the speech sound **s**, e.g. **nice**.

- Children may say **t** instead of **k**, for example **tar** instead of **car**. The speech sound **t** is made at the front of the mouth, by lifting the tip of the tongue and putting it behind the top teeth to stop the air coming out of the mouth. So **t** is a front sound and **k** is a back speech sound.

- If you tell the child to open their mouth as wide as they can and say **k**, the child cannot raise their tongue at the front of the mouth and say **t**.

- If you gently hold down the child's tongue at the front with a tongue depressor (ask your speech therapist to give you some or use unused wooden lollipop sticks), the child cannot raise their tongue at the front of the mouth and say **t**.

- Children may say **g** instead of **k**, for example **goat** instead of **coat**.

About this book

What is it?

Playing with k is a resource for nursery practitioners, teachers, teaching assistants, carers, speech and language therapists, and speech and language therapy assistants to use in helping children to say **k** in their talking. It contains activities, games and ideas to use with children aged from three to seven years. It can be used with older children who have learning difficulties. Each section contains simple, easy-to-follow instructions and practical tips to help you support the child you are working with. All of the materials can be photocopied and instructions are given to help you make the resources for activities. There are progress forms in each section to help you and the child record progress. There are also examples of session plans at the end to help you use the book.

Playing with k aims to:

- give children opportunities to hear **k** in games, activities and jingles

- give children opportunities to practise saying **k** in games, activities and jingles

- provide a clear, easy-to-follow structure for activities

- provide tips to help you support children who have difficulties with certain activities

- be fun!

How long should sessions be?

Keep sessions short and carry them out regularly, perhaps 15 minutes five days a week. Be flexible. For example, if the child is not able to concentrate for 15 minutes, perhaps if they have attention and listening difficulties, make sessions shorter and gradually lengthen them as and when the child is ready. If the child can concentrate for longer, you can increase the length of sessions. Every child is different and this book allows you to tailor sessions to suit the individual. Take sessions in a quiet environment so that the child can focus on the work that you are doing and will not be distracted.

How to use the book

The first seven sections follow the typical acquisition of speech sounds by children:

- Section 1 contains exercises for the mouth (oro-motor exercises). It aims to help children learn about their mouths and practise movements that can help speech, for example rounding and spreading their lips.

- Section 2 aims to help children say the single speech sound **k**.

- Section 3 contains short words that begin with the speech sound **k**, for example **car, key, cow.**

- Section 4 aims to help children say longer words that begin with the speech sound **k**, such as **can, comb, corn.**

- Section 5 contains words that end with the speech sound **k**, such as **duck, sock, book.**

- Section 6 contains words that begin with **k** and have more than one syllable, such as **cooker, kitten, coconut.**

- Section 7 provides opportunities to use all the words presented in the book in phrases and sentences.

Each activity section contains both listening and speaking activities. This gives the child opportunities to hear the speech sound and see how to say it before copying it in a speaking activity. For example: round your lips or spread your lips, raise your tongue at the front of the mouth or at the back of the mouth.

Sections 3, 4, 5 and 6 include sets of jingles and rhymes which use the words you have been working on with the child. For example: 'The **king can cook**. He **can cook** yummy **cakes**! The **queen can't**.'

At the end of each activity section you will find progress sheets to help you and the child record the progress you are making in the sessions.

Section 7 contains activities that can be used with the words from Sections 2, 3, 4, 5 and 6 to enable the child to say words in sentences.

Section 8 contains ideas for games that can be played using the words from Sections 2, 3, 4, 5 and 6. These provide the child with more opportunities to hear the words you are working on and to practise saying them. Instructions are given for each game. Templates for resources are included with instructions on how to make them.

There are examples of session plans in Section 9 to help you use the book.

This book allows you to be flexible and to follow the needs of the child that you are helping. The amount of time you work on each section will depend on the child and the speed of their progress. There are ideas for making the activities more challenging and tips on how to make them easier so that you can tailor what you are doing to suit each individual child.

You will see that Sections 3, 4, 5 and 6 contain some of the same activities, for example 'Listen and guess', 'What's the word?', but using different words. The activities use different words in different sections – short words in Section 3 (e.g. **car**, **key**, **core**), longer words that begin with **k** in Section 4 (e.g. **cup**, **comb**, **cake**), words that end with **k** in Section 5 (e.g. **duck**, **back**, **lake**) and words that begin with **k** and have more than one syllable in Section 6 (e.g. **kangaroo**, **carpet**, **coffee**). The activities have been printed in full in each section for the following reasons.

- All activities can be photocopied and used alone.

- You do not have to refer back to earlier sections in the book in order to find instructions for activities, although the tips in Section 3 will be helpful in later activities too.

- You can access the book easily at any level. For example, if the child you are working with is having difficulty saying **k** at the end of words, you can start working on Section 5 without having to look back to earlier sections for instructions.

Tip

Photocopy pictures and resources onto card or laminate them for all activities so that you can use them again. Cut out the small pictures of the words you are working on to use in activities and games.

How to help the child to use the speech sound in their everyday talking

Changing the way a child speaks can take time. This can be very frustrating for carers and the child. Using one speech sound instead of another, for example saying **t** in words instead of **k**, can become a habit. In order to change this habit, children need regular opportunities to hear the speech sound they are not yet using and to practise saying it.

Children are often able to use the speech sound they are working on, **k** in this case, in sessions with support from, say, a speech therapist or a teaching assistant. However, outside the sessions, they often continue to have difficulty using the speech sound in their talking. This can be demotivating for carers who are working with the child and for the child. Change does not happen overnight and progress can be slow. This is perfectly normal and does not mean the child will never be able to change their talking.

Using progress sheets will help you and the child to see progress. Tell older children that it will take time to help them say **k** in their talking and that you will need to work on saying **k** regularly. Photocopy exercises and activities from the book and give them to carers so that they can work with the child at home.

Tips

- Be careful not to overload the child as this can be demotivating! Keep sessions short and fun so that the child remains engaged and interested. Give lots of praise and positive feedback to encourage the child.

- Avoid correcting the child as this can make them feel bad about their talking and it does not help them to change the speech sounds they are using. Instead of correcting the child, repeat what they have said without the speech sound error so that the child has an opportunity to hear the word that they want to say but cannot yet say in their talking. For example: if the child says '**Tar**! A red **tar**!' you say '**Car**! A red **car**!' It can help the child if you repeat the word a few times in as natural a context as you can. For example: 'I can see a white **car**. We've got a white **car**, haven't we? Our **car** is a bit dirty. We can take it to a **car** wash' (four repetitions of **car**). This can feel unnatural and be difficult to do, but it is worth trying!

- The jingles at the end of sections give the child more opportunities to hear the words that you are working on. If possible, try reading them at set times, such as at bedtime or after dinner. As the jingles become more familiar and the child makes progress with their talking, start leaving pauses for them to complete the jingles. For example: 'The king can _____ (**cook**)'. (See the instructions for using jingles at the end of Section 3.)

- Encourage children to think about their talking so that they are actively involved in the speech therapy work. Give them information about speech sounds to help them monitor their talking. For example: 'You said **tar**. We make t at the front of the mouth. Look!' [Use a mirror to show the child that your tongue lifts at the front of the mouth to say **t**.] 'I said car. We make k at the back of the mouth. Look!' [Use a mirror to show the child that your tongue lifts at the back of the mouth to say **k**.] This can help children to listen and learn more about the speech sound they actually say and the speech sound they want to say. Often children do not know that they are saying, for example, **t** instead of **k** in words. They need your help and support to realise that what they are saying is not what they want to say. Always model a speech sound or word for children so that they can hear it before they try to say it. Help older children to reflect on what they say. For example: 'I said car. You said tar. Are they the same? Listen. **Car. Tar.**' Raise their awareness by offering them choices. For example: 'Is it **tar** [hold out a fist as you say **tar**] or is it car [hold out the other fist]?' If the child cannot yet say **k** in words, they can choose between **car** and **tar** by touching one of your fists, either the fist that you held out when you said **tar**, or the fist that you held out when you said **car**.

How to use this book in the nursery or the classroom

- Play group or class listening games at carpet time – after registration, before break times, after lunch. You could put one of the resources to help children say **k** on the board, for example 'Put a cat on a cushion and say k' from Section 2. Choose a child to come to the board. Ask the child to listen and when they hear you say **k**, put a cat on a cushion. Count silently to at least four before you say **k** so that the child has to wait. When the child has finished their go, ask them to choose another child to come to the board to listen and put a cat on a cushion when they hear **k**. Let the first child say **k** for the second child. The children take it in turns to choose the next child to be the listener and to say **k** in the activity (see the listening activities in Section 2).

- See the instructions for games using words containing the speech sound **k** in Section 8, for example charades. Play these with the group or class perhaps before lunch or at the end of the day before home time.

- Choose a word of the week from the words you have been working on. Put it on the board and tell the group or class that they have to clap or stand up every time they hear you say the word.

- Get a feely bag. Instead of pictures of the words you have been working on, find objects, such as a key, a toy cow, a toy car. Put one in the bag. Look in the bag and describe the object to the children. For example: 'It's an animal. It lives on a farm. It eats grass and we get milk from it. It says moo, moo! Hands up if you know what it is!' Put one object in the bag. Pass it to a child. The child feels the object through the bag, without looking, and guesses what it is. Change the object and give the bag to the next child.

- Read at least one jingle from the jingle sections in this book to the group or class. See the instructions on ideas for using the jingles at the end of Section 3.

- Have a 'jingle of the week' and teach the children actions to go with it to make the jingle more memorable and fun!

- Make your own jingles in class using curriculum vocabulary words that contain **k**.

- Start a **k** poster in the class. When you work on curriculum topic vocabulary such as mini beasts, habitats, our environment, put words that contain **k** on the poster (with pictures if possible to make them more visual).

- Play mouth exercise games with the group or class at carpet time or before literacy sessions. See Section 1 of this book for activities, games and pictures.

Tip

- Photocopy resources and give them to carers so they can work with the child at home.

Author's note

Sections 3, 4, 5 and 6 include some activities which are the same but carried out with different words. These have been written out in full each time so they can be photocopied easily, to avoid having to refer back to instructions in an earlier section and so that the resource can be accessed from any section. For example, if the child is having difficulty saying **k** at the end of words, you can start from Section 5.

SECTION 1

EXERCISES FOR THE MOUTH

Section 1: Exercises for the mouth

Aim
To learn about our mouths and practise movements that can help speech.

How?
By giving the child opportunities to see you carry out the exercises and to copy them.

Resources
*   A mirror so that the child can watch herself copying the exercises.

*   Large pictures of mouth exercises (pp. 14–25).

*   At least two sets of small pictures of mouth exercises (p.26–27) with shapes on the back (p. 28) (photocopy the sheet of shapes onto the back of one set of small pictures so that the pictures are double-sided) and at least two sets of small pictures without shapes on the back.

*   A dice (p. 29).

*   The template for a dice with a different shape on each face (p. 30).

*   A copy of the resource that tells you how to speak, e.g. Say it in a quiet voice, Say it in a loud voice, Say it in a sad voice (p. 181).

Instructions
1   Put the mirror in front of the child so that you can see yourselves. Tell the child that you are going to do some exercises for your mouth! Before you start, ask her, for example, to show you her tongue; show you her teeth; open her mouth wide; give you a big smile. Encourage her to look in the mirror when she does these warm-up movements.

2   Look at the large pictures, read the instruction and demonstrate the movement for the child using the mirror. Then say 'You try!'

Note: the instruction 'smile like a granny' means to smile without showing your teeth (i.e. spread your lips).

Keep this activity short and fun.

Variations
When the child is familiar with the exercises, make them more challenging:
*   Carry out the instructions to do a sequence of movements, e.g. *Can you put your tongue up to your nose and then down to your chin?* Always demonstrate movements for the child before she has a turn, so that she can see what you want her to do.

- Take it in turns to roll the dice and carry out the sequence of movements that number of times. For example, if the child throws a four, she has to move her tongue up and down four times.

- Turn the set of small pictures face down on the table so that you can see the shapes on the back but not the pictures of the mouth movement. Use the template to make a dice with shapes on the faces. Take it in turns to throw the shape dice at least twice. Turn over the pictures that have those shapes on the back. If you throw a circle, turn over the picture that has a circle on it so that you can see the picture of the mouth movement, e.g. *smile like a granny*. If you throw a star, turn over the picture that has a star on it so that you can see the picture of the mouth movement, e.g. *say **ee***. Then throw the number dice to see how many times you have to do the mouth movements. For example: if you throw a 6, you have to smile like a granny and then say **ee** six times.

- Put at least two sets of the small pictures (without the shapes on the back) face down in front of the child. Take it in turns to turn over two pictures and do the movement on each picture. If the two pictures are the same, for example *blow a kiss* and *blow a kiss*, keep them as a pair. The winner is the person who has the most pairs.

- Photocopy the resource that tells you how to speak, e.g. *say it in a quiet voice*, *say it in a happy voice*, and cut it into cards. Put them in a pile, face down. Put at least two sets of the small picture pictures of *say ah*, *say oo* and *say ee* face down in front of the child. Take it in turns to turn a picture over, e.g. *say **oo***, and take a picture from the other pile, e.g. say it in a loud voice. Carry out the instructions. For example, if one picture is *say **oo*** and the other is *say it in a loud voice*, you have to say the speech sound **oo** loudly!

- Place a barrier between you and the child so that you cannot see each other's pictures. Make sure that you both have at least two sets of the small pictures of mouth movements. Choose at least four pictures from your set. For example: *smile like a granny, blow a kiss, smile like a granny, say ee*. Do not show the child. Arrange the pictures behind the barrier so that she cannot see them. The child then watches you copy the mouth movements on the pictures you have put behind the barrier and puts the matching pictures from her set behind the barrier. When she has finished, ask her to show you the mouth movements that are on the pictures she has chosen so that she has a turn at copying the movements. Then remove the barrier to see if she has the same pictures as you. When the child is familiar with this activity, reverse it so that she chooses the pictures and demonstrates them for you.

My progress

Date	I can ...	☺/☹	I need to work on ...
	Do all of the mouth exercises without any help.		
	Do all of the mouth exercises with some help.		
	Do most of the mouth exercises without any help.		
	Do most of the mouth exercises with some help.		
	Do some of the mouth exercises without any help.		
	Do some of the mouth exercises with some help.		
	Do a few of the mouth exercises without any help.		
	Do a few of the mouth exercises with some help.		

Tips

To practise lip movements:

- Try blowing whistles, blowing kisses, blowing bubbles, blowing musical instruments, whistling!

- Put on lipstick and kiss a piece of paper – one for the girls!

- Fill cheeks with air and then pop!

To practise tongue movements:

- Try holding a small food item, e.g. a Cheerio or a Polo, on the skin just behind the top teeth (alveolar ridge). Tell the child to push against it as hard as he can with his tongue.

- Gently touch around the child's mouth, e.g. his chin, one of his cheeks, his nose. The child has to move his tongue to the place you touched.

- Put your tongue inside your cheek and push against the child's cheek! Try pushing back against the child's tongue so that he has to push harder.

smile like a granny 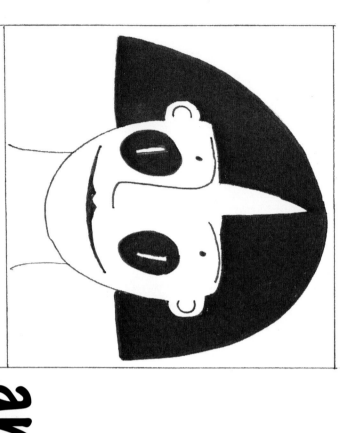 and then

say oo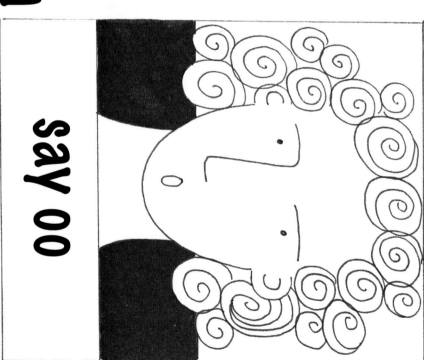

can you

can you

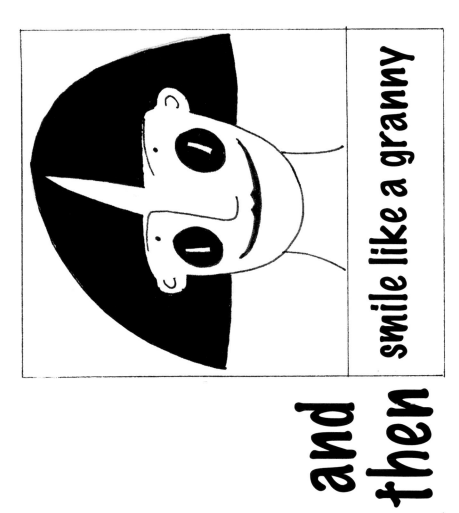

smile like a granny

and
then

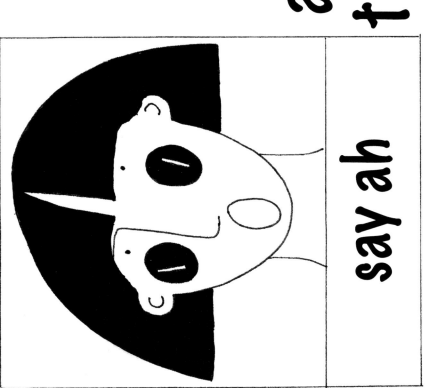

say ah

can you put your tongue

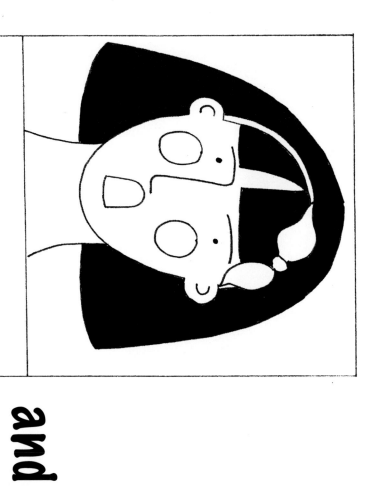

up to your nose

and then

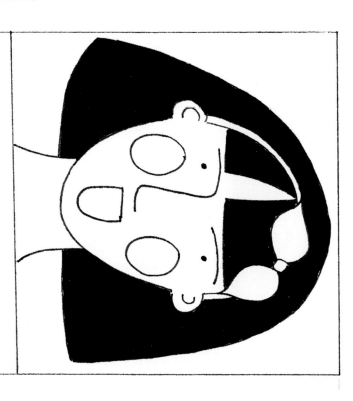

down to your chin

16

can you

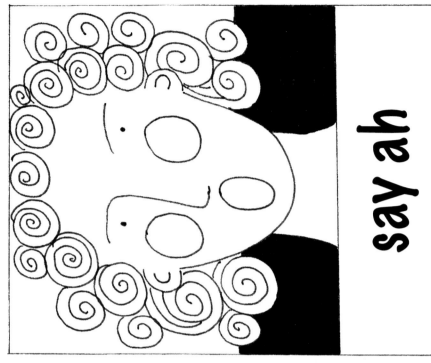

say ah

and
then

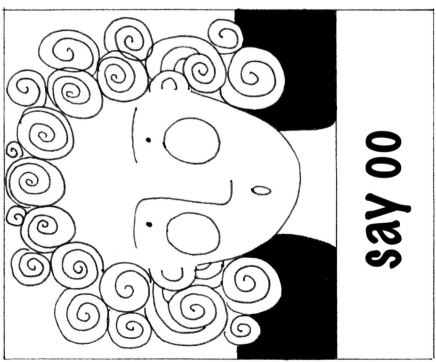

say oo

blow a kiss

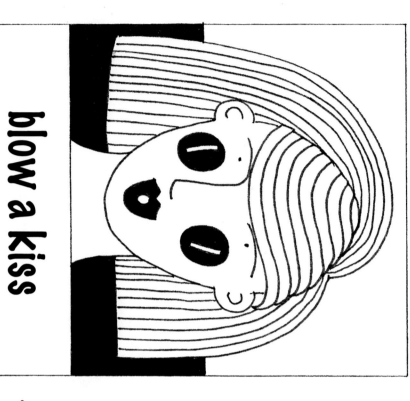

and then

smile like a granny

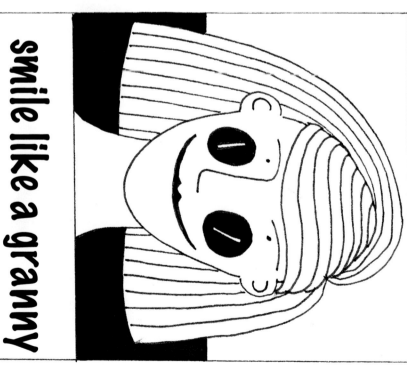

can you

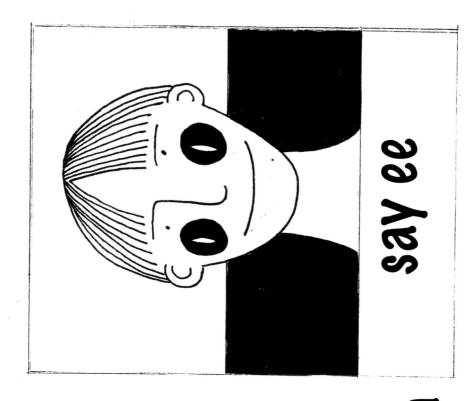

say ee

and
then

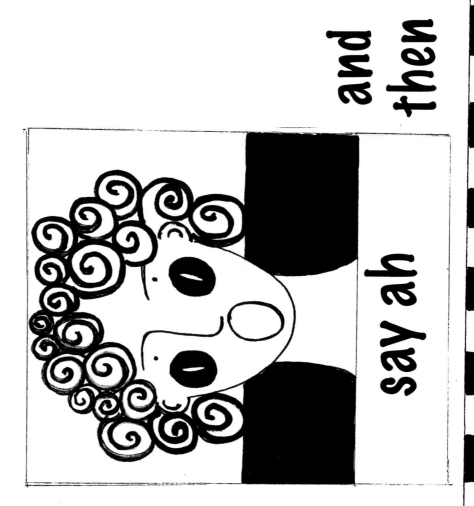

say ah

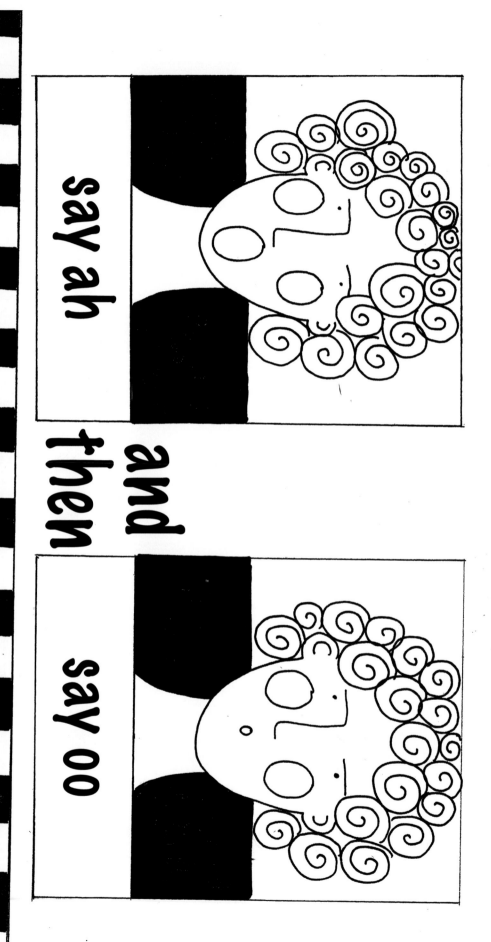

can you

say ah

and then

say oo

can you put your tongue

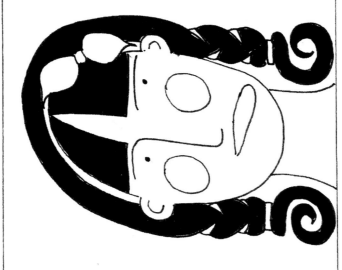

right

and
then

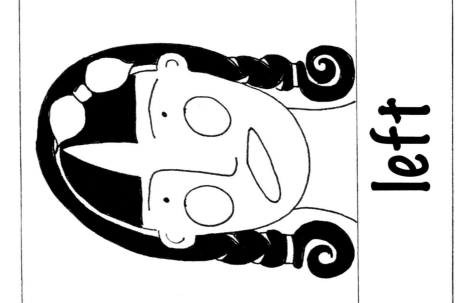

left

can you put your tongue

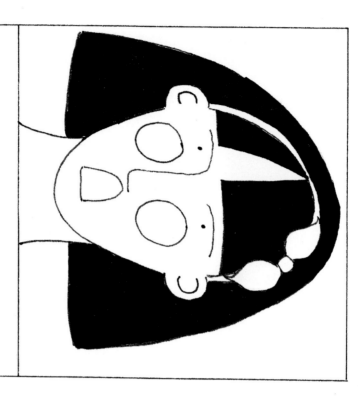

up to your nose

and
then

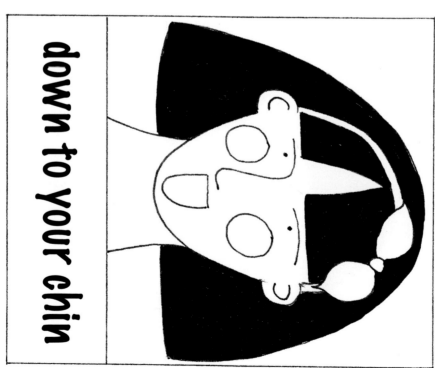

down to your chin

can you put your tongue

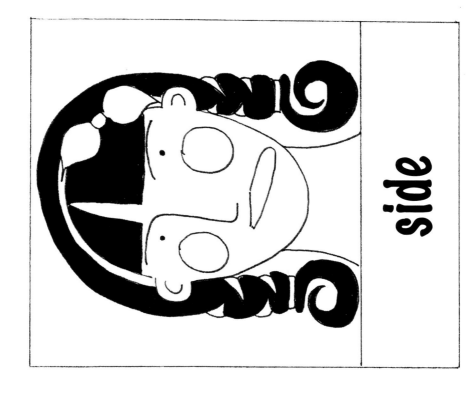

side

to

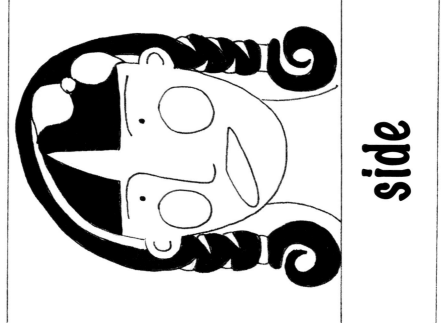

side

can you

fill your cheeks with air

and then

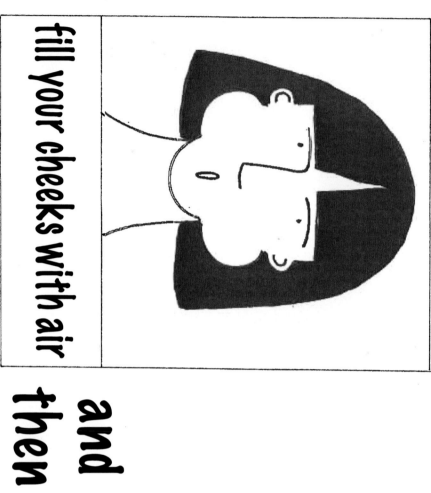

pop your cheeks!

can you

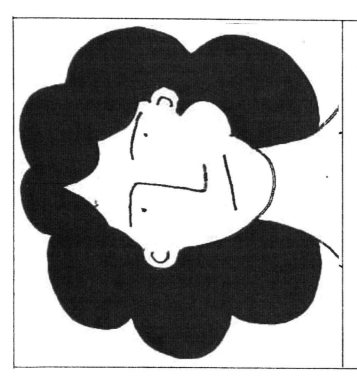

push against your cheek
with your tongue

and
then

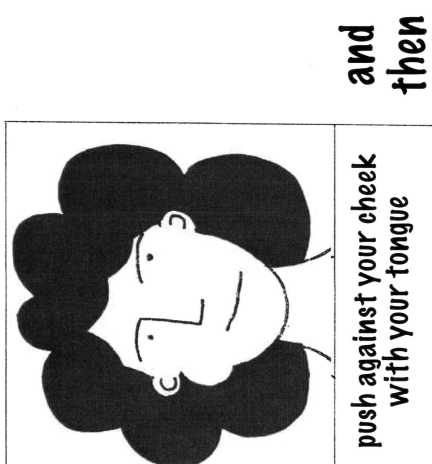

push against your cheek
with your tongue

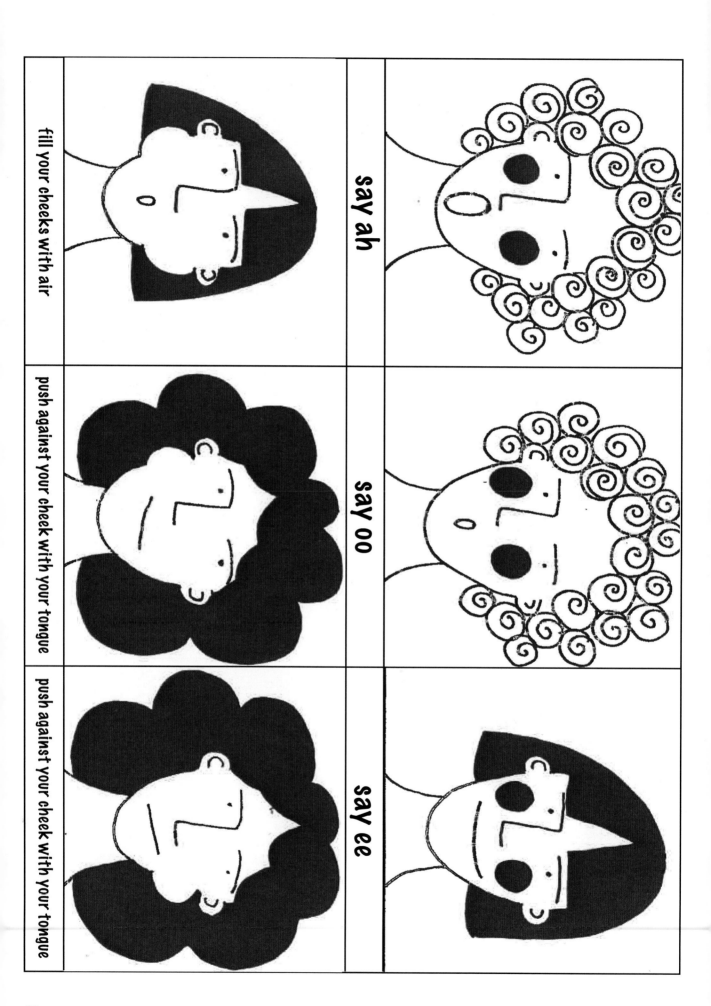

say ah

say oo

say ee

fill your cheeks with air

push against your cheek with your tongue

push against your cheek with your tongue

26

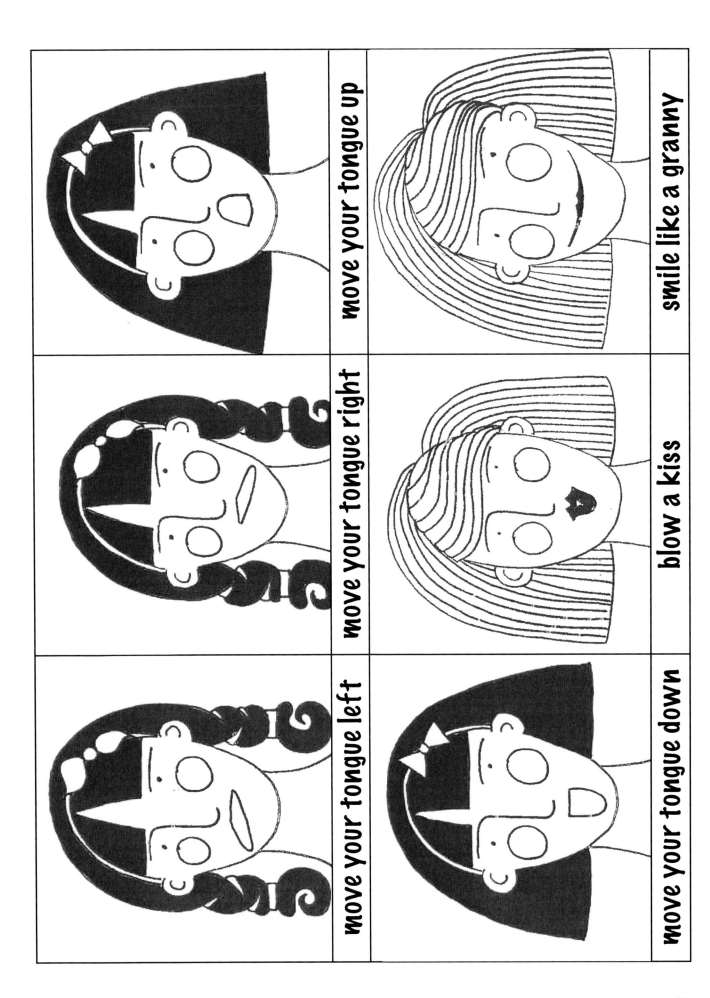

move your tongue up

smile like a granny

move your tongue right

blow a kiss

move your tongue left

move your tongue down

27

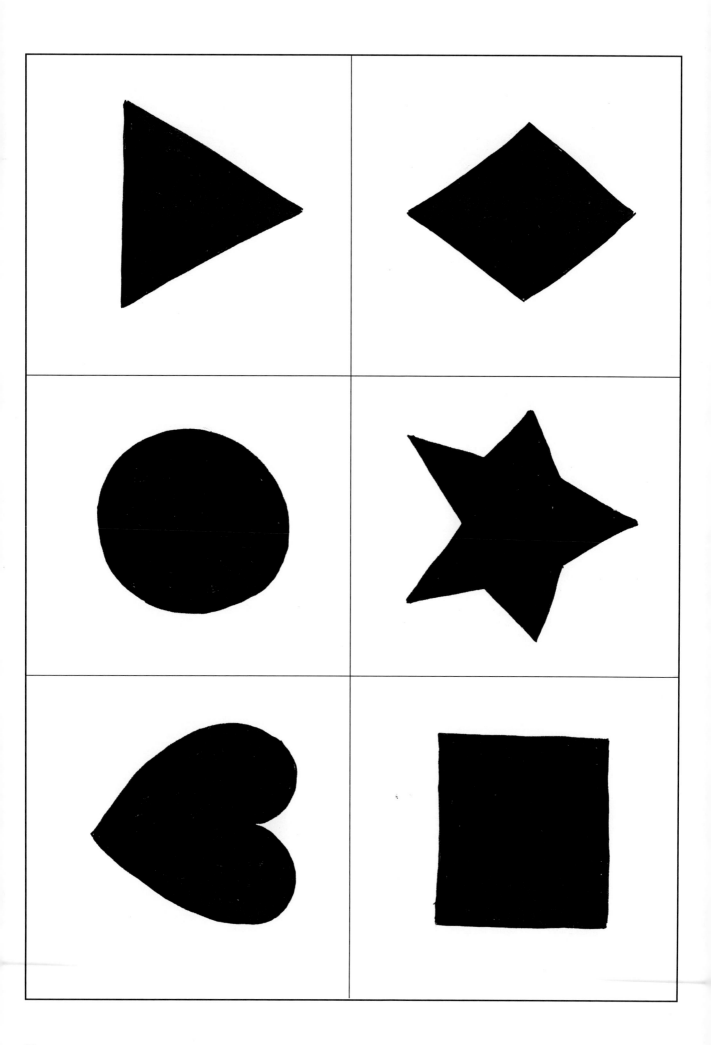

Template for a dice

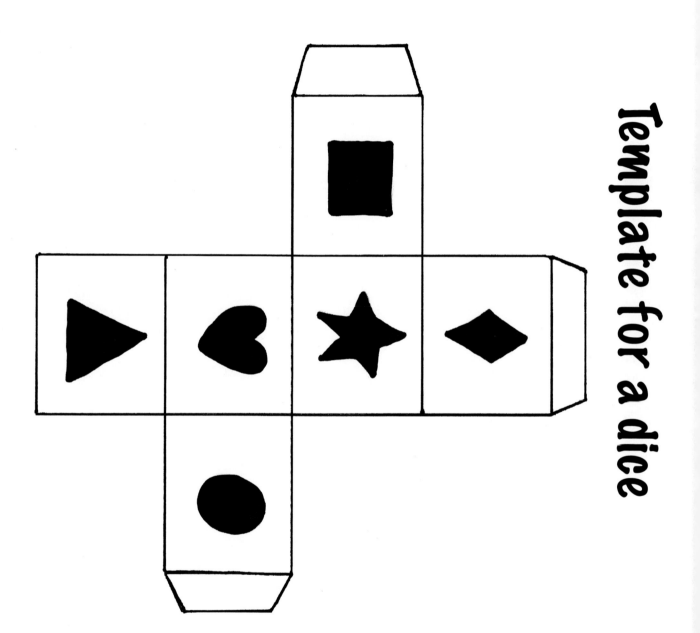

Template for a dice

SECTION 2
SAYING K

PLAYING WITH K

32

Section 2 Saying k

Saying the speech sound k (1) (Listening and speaking activity)

Aim

To say the speech sound **k**.

How?

By giving the child opportunities to hear, and see, you say **k** and to copy you.

Resources

- Picture of nine cats and three cushions (p. 44). Photocopy the page twice. Laminate one page and put small pieces of Velcro or Blu-Tack on each of the cats, and three small pieces of Velcro or Blu-Tack on each cushion. Cut out the line of cats from the other page and laminate it. Cut out the cats and put a small piece of Velcro or Blu-Tack on the back of each cat. Stick each cat on top of a cat on the picture of cats and cushions.

- Picture of crowns and kings (p. 45). Photocopy the page twice. Laminate one page and put small pieces of Velcro or Blu-Tack on each of the crowns and on each king's head. Cut out the line of crowns from the other page and laminate it. Cut out the crowns and put a small piece of Velcro or Blu-Tack on the back of each crown. Stick each crown on top of a crown in the picture of kings and crowns.

- Pictures of nine candles and three cakes (p. 46). Photocopy the page twice. Laminate one page and put small pieces of Velcro or Blu-Tack on each of the candles, and three small pieces of Velcro or Blu-Tack on each cake. Cut out the line of candles from the other page and laminate it. Cut out the candles and put a small piece of Velcro or Blu-Tack on the back of each candle. Stick each candle on top of a candle on the picture of candles and cakes.

Instructions

1 Read the instruction at the top of the page to the child: *Put a **cat** on a **cushion** and say k*. Before you carry out the instruction, say: 'My turn!' so that the child knows you are going to do the task first. Then take a cat, stick it on a cushion and say **k**. (Remember to say the speech sound **k**, not the letter **k** (kay). See 'The speech sound k' in the Introduction.)

2 When you have finished your go, say: 'Your turn!' so that the child knows it is his go. The child takes a cat, puts it on a cushion and says **k**. Take turns until all the cats are on the cushions, all the crowns are on the kings, and all the candles are on the cakes.

Variations

Listening activities

- Tell the child to listen carefully and to put a cat on a cushion when you say **k**. Count silently to at least four and then say **k**. When the child hears you say **k**, he takes a cat and puts it on a cushion. If the child finds this activity hard, demonstrate it on a toy or a puppet. For example, tell the toy or the puppet to listen and put a cat on a cushion when you say **k**. This gives the child an opportunity to watch the activity before he has a go. It also helps to reduce any feelings of anxiety he might have about taking part in the activity.

- To make this listening activity harder, again ask the child to listen carefully and put a cat on a cushion when you say **k** but this time say at least four other speech sounds before you say **k**, e.g. **m**, **s**, **p**, **sh**, **k**. Leave pauses between each speech sound to help the child listen for **k**.

- Try reversing the activity so that the child asks you, or the puppet or toy, to listen and put a cat on a cushion when he says **k**.

Speaking activities

See how many times in a minute the child can put a cat on a cushion and say **k**. Use a one-minute salt timer to time him.

Saying the speech sound k (2) (Listening and speaking activity)

Aim

To say the speech sound **k**.

How?

By giving the child opportunities to hear, and see, you say **k** and to copy you.

Resources

- Template for a speech sound dice (p. 40).

- Hand prints to photocopy (p. 41).

- Heads, without hair, to photocopy (p. 43).

- Aliens to photocopy (p. 42).

- Coloured pencils or pens.

Instructions

1 Make a dice using the template. If the child cannot say any of the speech sounds on the template (**m, n, w, d, t, h**), use a blank template and write speech sounds that the child can say on it. For instance, you could put three speech sounds instead of six, e.g. **m, m, n, n, t, t**.

2 Choose a template to photocopy for the activity, e.g. colouring rings on fingers, drawing hair on a head. Photocopy the sheet.

3 Roll the dice to choose a speech sound, e.g. **m**.

4 Choose two colour pencils, e.g. orange and blue. Say the speech sound **k** and draw a strand of hair on one of the heads. Change colour pencils, say the speech sound that you rolled on the dice, e.g. **m**, and draw a second strand of hair on the head. Repeat this ten times so that you draw five orange hairs and say **k** five times, and five blue hairs and say **m** five times.

5 Take turns to say the two speech sounds and draw a hair on the head (or colour in a ring, or draw an eye on the alien).

Variations

- Use the activities as listening games, e.g. 'When I say **k**, colour in a ring.'

- Use the activities to practise saying **k**. For example, take it in turns to say **k** and colour in a ring.

- Say **k** and draw a strand of hair on a head. Change colours and say the speech sound you rolled on the dice, e.g. **m**, and draw another strand of hair. The child then says **k** and draws a strand of hair on the same head, changes colour, and says the speech sound you rolled on the dice, e.g. **m**, and draws another strand of hair. Take it in turns until you have drawn at least twelve strands of hair on the head and said the speech sounds six times each.

- Take it in turns to say the two speech sounds, e.g. **k** and **m**, six times, drawing strands of hair on the head after you have said each one. When you and the child have both had a go, there should be twelve strands of hair on the head.

Tip

*Help! The child says **t** instead of **k**! What can I do?*

- Children often say **t** instead of **k**. For example, they might say **tar** instead of **car**. Developmentally, children say **t** before they say **k**. The speech sound **t** is made at the front of the mouth, by lifting the tip of the tongue and putting it behind the top teeth to stop the air coming out of the mouth. The speech sound **t** is a front sound and the speech sound **k** is a back sound. Use a mirror to show the child how to say **k** and how to say **t** so that he can see the difference. We say **k** by lifting the back of the tongue to touch the roof of the mouth and block the air from coming out of the mouth. If you tell the child to open his mouth as wide as he can and say **k**, the child's tongue cannot lift at the front of his mouth, so he cannot say **t**.

- Before you ask the child to open his mouth as wide as he can, show him how wide you can open your mouth! Use a mirror so you can both see how wide you can open your mouth! Then ask the child if he can open his mouth as wide as you can! Say 'Look what I can do!', open your mouth as wide as you can and say **k**. Then ask the child if he can do that.

- If you gently but firmly hold the child's tongue down at the front with a tongue depressor (ask your speech and language therapist to give you some or use unused wooden lollipop sticks), the child cannot raise his tongue at the front of the mouth and say **t**. Many children find this very intrusive and do not like having a tongue depressor put in their mouths. It can seem very clinical and be unsettling for the child. I don't want to put you off trying this approach, as it can be very successful, but be warned:

  - If you put the tongue depressor too far back in the child's mouth, you can make the child gag.

  - If you hold the tongue tip down too lightly when you ask the child to say **k**, he will lift it to say **t** as it has become a habit to say **t** instead of **k**.

  - This approach can put a child off trying to say **k**, so if the child does not respond well to it, stop.

  Ask your speech therapist for help if you are worried about using a tongue depressor.

- A sense of humour always helps and demonstrating it on yourself or on a toy can help reduce the child's anxiety.

- Lying on his back on the floor can make it easier for the child to lift the back of the tongue instead of the front. It is also a bit silly, so children usually love it!

- Try giving the child more information about the speech sound **k**. For example: 'You said **t**. That's a front sound. Look at my mouth when I say **t**. Am I lifting the back of my tongue or the front? That's right, I'm lifting the front of my tongue. Look again: **t**, **t**, **t**. I said **t**. That's a front sound. Look at my mouth when I say **k**. Am I lifting the back of my tongue or the front? That's right, I'm lifting the back of my tongue. Look: **k**, **k**, **k**.'

*Help! The child says **g** instead of **k**! What can I do?*

- Give the child more information about the speech sound he said, e.g. **g**, and the one you wanted him to say, e.g. **k**. For example: 'You said **g**. That's a noisy sound. Listen: **g**, **g**, **g**. I said **k**. That's a quiet sound. Listen: **k**, **k**, **k**.'

- Try asking the child to whisper **k**. Sometimes children can whisper **k**, but when they try to say **k** in a louder voice, they say **g**.

- Say 'Copy me!' to the child. Whisper **k** at least five times, e.g. '**k**, **k**, **k**, **k**, **k**.' Then say 'Your turn!' and the child whispers **k** five times. Say 'My turn!' and whisper **k** five times again, but make sure the fifth time you say **k** you say it a little bit louder than the other four. Each session, see if you can make the fifth **k** just a fraction louder until the child is saying **k** quietly.

My progress

Date	I can ...	☺/☹	I need to work on ...
	Listen carefully and put a cat on a cushion when I hear **k** without any help.		
	Listen carefully and put a cat on a cushion when I hear **k** with help.		
	Listen carefully to different speech sounds, e.g. **m**, **s**, **p**, **sh**, **k**, and put a cat on a cushion when I hear **k** without any help.		
	Listen carefully to different speech sounds, e.g. **m**, **s**, **p**, **sh**, **k**, and put a cat on a cushion when I hear **k** with help.		
	Say **k** without any help.		
	Say **k** with help.		
	Say **k** with other speech sounds, e.g. I can say **m**, **k**, **m**, **k**, **m**, **k**, **m**, **k**, without any help.		
	Say **k** with other speech sounds, e.g. I can say **m**, **k**, **m**, **k**, **m**, **k**, **m**, **k**, with help.		

What's the next step?

- I can listen carefully and put a cat on a cushion when I say **k** without any help. I can listen carefully to different speech sounds, e.g. **m**, **s**, **p**, **sh**, **k**, and put a cat on a cushion when I hear **k** without any help. **Start listening activities in Section 3.**

- I can listen carefully and put a cat on a cushion when I hear **k** with help. I can listen carefully to different speech sounds, e.g. **m**, **s**, **p**, **sh**, **k**, and put a cat on a cushion when I hear **k** with help. **Continue playing listening games from Section 2, but start to gradually include listening games from Section 3.**

- I can say **k** without any help. I can say **k** with other speech sounds, e.g. I can say **m**, **k**, **m**, **k**, **m**, **k**, **m**, **k**, without any help. **Start Section 3 saying k at the beginning of short words, e.g. car, key, cow.**

- I can say **k** with help. I can say **k** with other speech sounds, e.g. I can say **m**, **k**, **m**, **k**, **m**, **k**, **m**, **k**, with help. **Continue working on activities in Section 2 to practise saying k and doing mouth exercises from Section 1.**

When the child can say k at least 70 per cent of the time, gradually introduce activities from Section 3.

Tips

- To work out if the child can say **k** at least 70 per cent of the time, listen to him saying **k** ten times, e.g. saying **k** and colouring in a ring ten times, or saying **k** and drawing an eye on an alien ten times. If he says **k** correctly seven out of ten times, he has said **k** 70 per cent of the time.

- The 70 per cent is a guideline to help you progress through the sections in this book. You know the child you are working with and there might be times when you think he is ready to move on and start the next section before he is able to say **k** 70 per cent of the time. For example, he might be able to say **k** 65 per cent of the time, or you might be concerned that he is losing interest in the words he is working on.

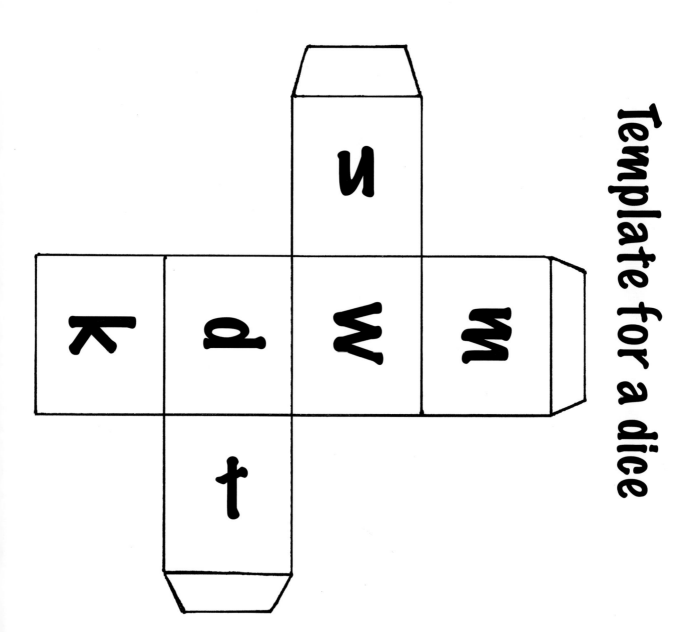

Template for a dice

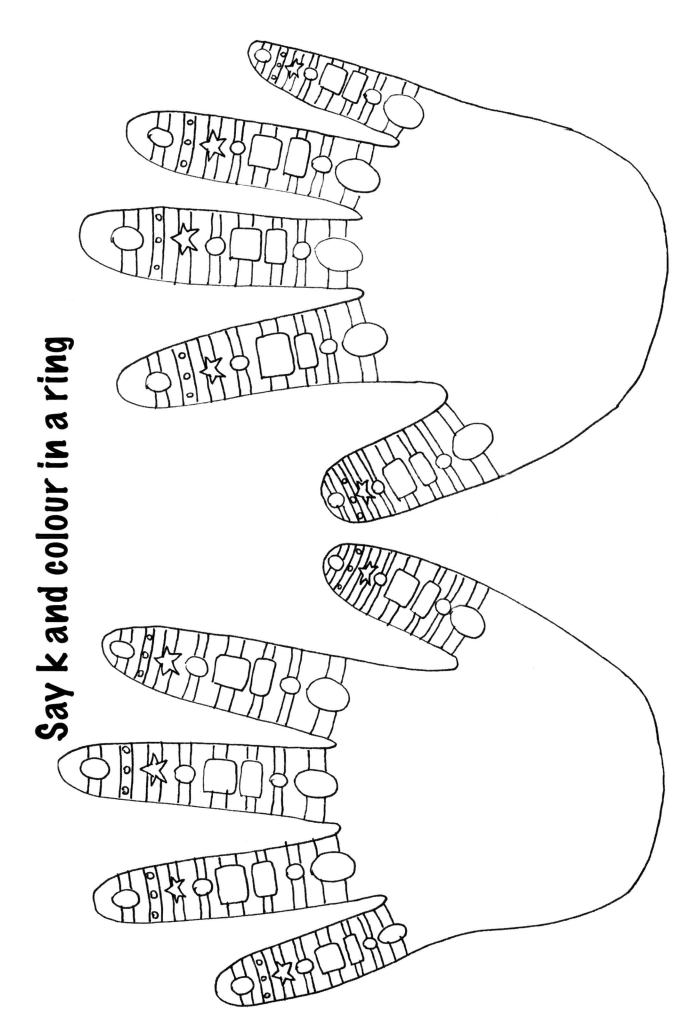

Say k and colour in a ring

41

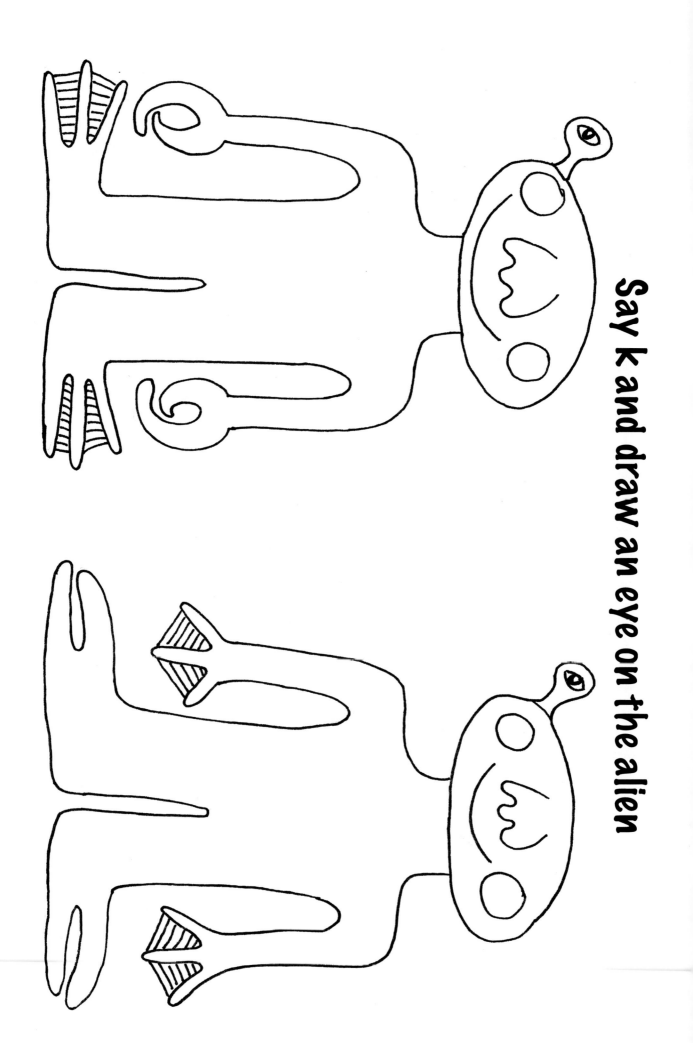

Say k and draw an eye on the alien

Say k and draw a strand of hair on a head

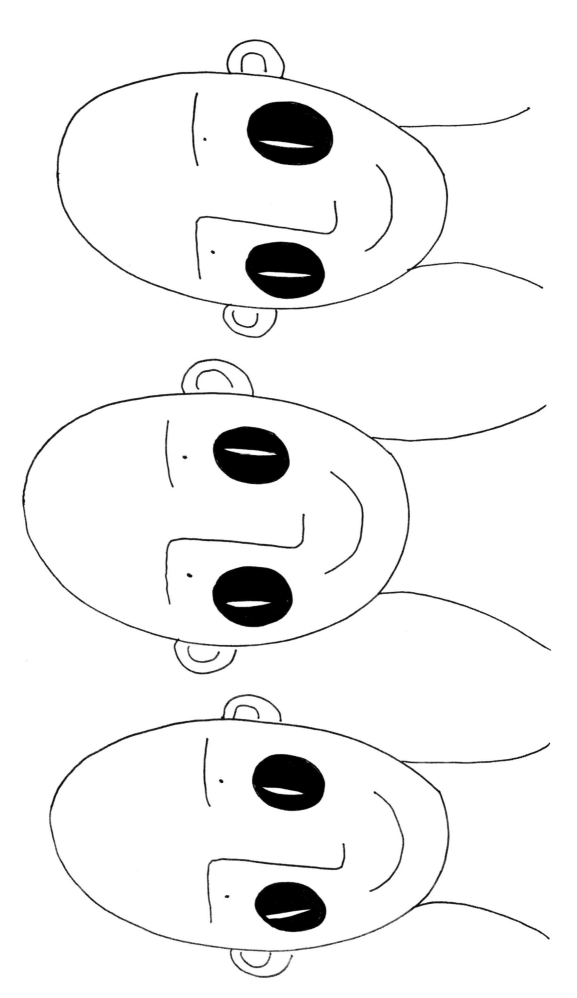

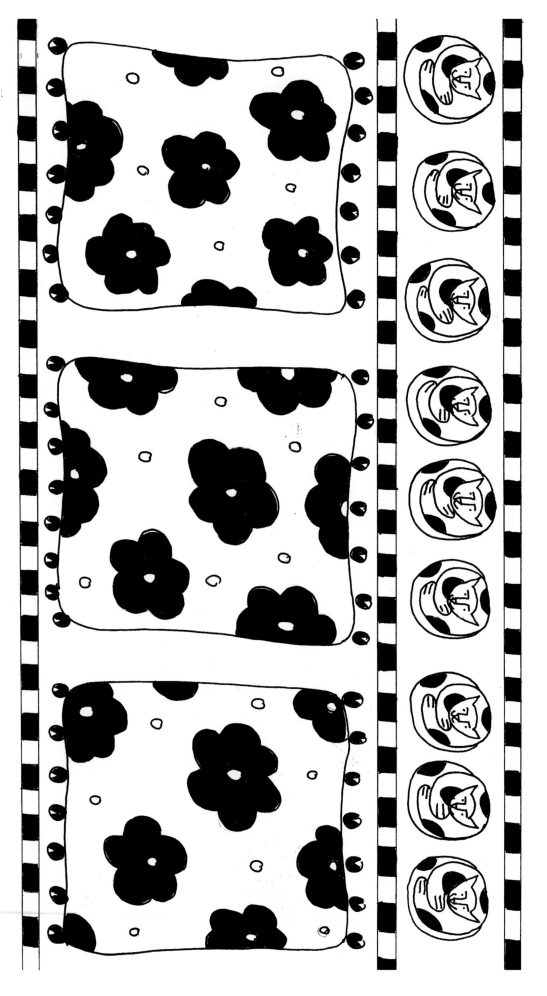

Put a cat on a cushion and say k

Put a crown on a king and say k

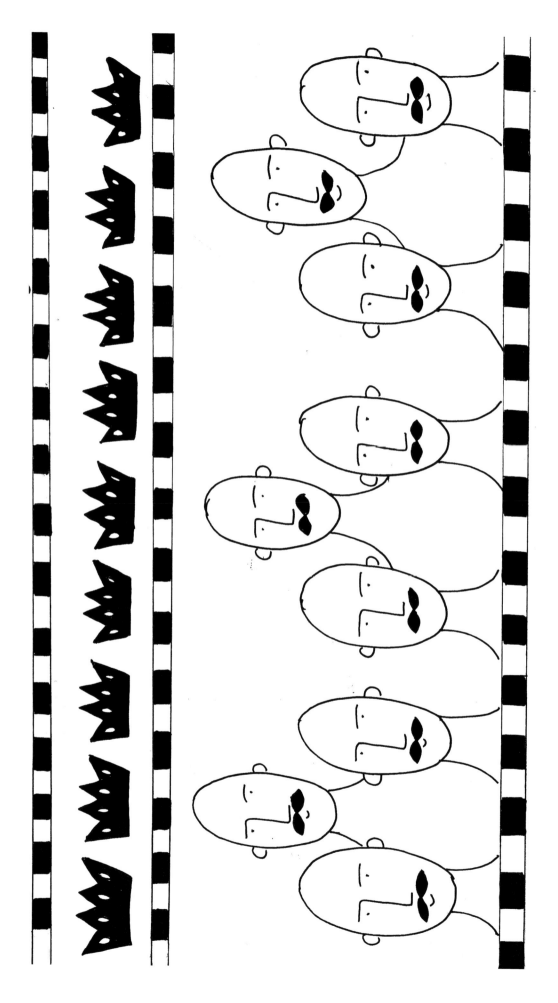

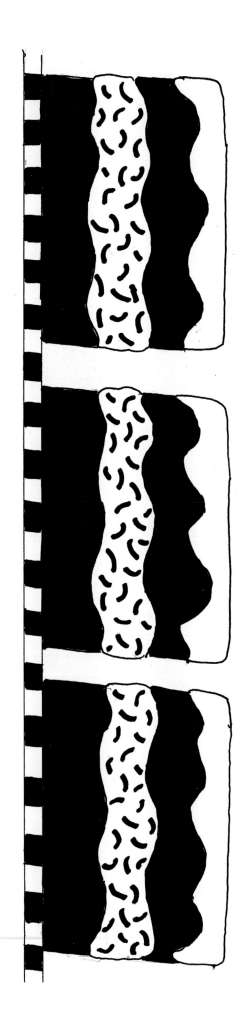

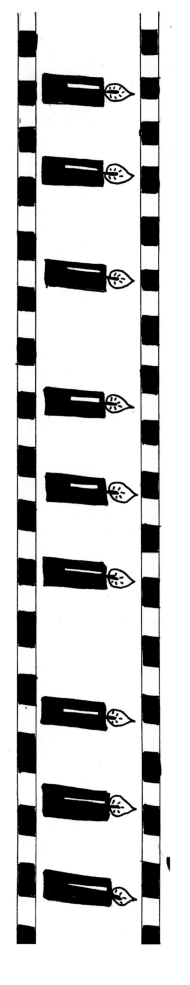

Put a candle on a cake and say k

SECTION 3

SAYING K AT THE BEGINNING OF SHORT WORDS

Section 3: Saying k at the beginning of short words

What's the picture? (Speaking activity)

Aim
To say short words that begin with the speech sound **k**: **key**, **car**, **core**, **cow**, **Kai**, **Kay**.

How?
By giving the child opportunities to hear, and see, you say short words that begin with **k** and to practise saying the words.

Resources
- Large pictures of short words that begin with **k** (pp. 59–61).

- Small pictures of short words that begin with **k** (p. 58).

- Page of two doors with question marks on each one and the instruction *What's the picture?* (p. 62). You will need to photocopy this page and cut along three sides of the doors so that you can open them to reveal a picture.

Instructions
1 Put the page with the doors on top of large pictures of words that begin with **k**, e.g. **car** and **key**.

2 Read the instruction at the top of the page to the child: *What's the picture? Open the door and see!* Before you open the door to see what the picture is, say: 'My turn!' so that the child knows you are going first. Open the first door to reveal the picture and name it, e.g. 'Look! **Car**!' so that the child has an opportunity to hear you say **k** at the beginning of a short word.

3 When you have finished your go, say to the child: 'Your turn!' so that she knows that it is her go to open the door and name the picture behind it.

4 Put the picture of the doors over different large pictures, e.g. **core** and **cow**, and take it in turns to open a door and name the picture behind it. Follow this procedure to name all the large pictures on the pages for this activity.

Variation
- Tell the child to close her eyes and put a small picture of a word beginning with **k** behind each door. Then ask the child to open her eyes and open the doors. Try asking her to guess which picture is behind the door before she opens it.

Tips

*Help! The child says **tar** instead of **car**. What can I do?*

- Don't expect the child to be able to say **k** in words immediately. Give her plenty of opportunities to hear words that begin with **k**. You could try to use the words you are working on several times in conversation, e.g. 'Look! **Car**! I've got a **car**. My **car** is very small and it is always very dirty! My children clean the **car** if I give them a lot of sweets!'

- See the advice in Section 2 for helping children to say **k**.

- If the child can say **k** most of the time, e.g. 70 per cent of the time, break the word into two parts, e.g. **k** + **ar**. Say the two parts, leaving a pause between them: **k** (pause) – **ar**. Put two fingers on the table in a V shape, touch the first finger when you say **k** and touch the second finger when you say **ar**. Ask the child to copy you. Gradually make the pause shorter and bring your fingers closer together until your fingers are touching and there is no pause between **k** and **ar**: i.e. you are saying **car**.

Help! The child won't try to say the words because she thinks she will make mistakes. What can I do?

- If the child gets anxious in activities and games, or is very unconfident, try using a puppet or a toy in sessions to reduce stress for her. Carry out the activities with the puppet or toy so that the child can watch and listen, but is not under any pressure to talk.

Note: These tips can also help you work on the words in Sections 4, 5 and 6.

Hide the cat (Speaking and listening activity)

Aim

To hear and say the speech sound **k** at the beginning of short words: **key, car, core, cow, Kai, Kay**.

How?

By giving the child opportunities to hear, and see, you say short words that begin with **k** and to practise saying the words.

Resources

- Large pictures of short words that begin with **k** (pp. 59–61).

- Small pictures of short words that begin with **k** (p. 58).

- Page of two doors with question marks on each one and the instruction *Close your eyes!* (p. 63). You will need to photocopy this page and cut along three sides of the doors so that you can open them to reveal a picture.

- A laminated picture of a cat with a small piece of Velcro or Blu-Tack on the back.

Instructions

1. Look at the pictures with the child: 'Look! A **cat**, a **key** and a **car**.' Read the first part of the instruction at the top of the doors page: *Close your eyes. I'm going to hide the **cat**!* Then stick the cat on the picture of the key or on the picture of the car and put the door over it. Read the rest of the instruction to the child: *Open your eyes! Where's the **cat**?* The child has to name the picture that she thinks the **cat** is on, e.g. '**Key**', and then open the door to see if she is right or not. Play this game several times, varying the pictures that you use.

2. Reverse the game. Say to the child: 'Your turn. I'll close my eyes and you hide the **cat**!' Let the child have several turns at hiding the cat. To ensure that the child does not get to know which picture to expect, put a small picture behind each door rather than putting the doors over a page of pictures.

Variations

- If the child finds this activity hard, play it as a listening game. For example, tell the child to close her eyes. Hide the cat on one of the pictures, e.g. **cow**. Tell the child to open her eyes and then you tell her where the cat is:

  'Turn your listening ears on! Are you ready? The **cat** is on the **cow**.' Use a toy or puppet to play this with younger children. Tell the toy or puppet where the cat is and the child helps the toy or puppet find it.

- Show the child at least two of the small pictures, e.g. **Kay** and **core**. Name the pictures. Ask the child to close her eyes. Put a **cat** under one of the small pictures. Ask the child to open her eyes and ask her 'Where's the **cat**?' The child names the picture that she thinks the cat is under, e.g. '**core**', and looks under the picture to see if she is right or not.

- Show the child at least four small pictures and name them, e.g. '**Kay. key. core. Kai.**' Then tell the child you are going to hide two **cats**! Ask her to close her eyes while you put a cat under two of the pictures. Ask the child to open her eyes and ask her 'Where are the **cats**?' The child names the pictures that she thinks a cat is under, e.g. '**Kay** and **Kai**', and looks to see if she is right or not. You can increase the number of pictures and the number of cats in the game. Remember to give the child a turn at hiding a cat for you to find.

What did I say? (Listening and speaking activity)

Aim
To say short words that begin with the speech sound **k**: **key**, **car**, **core**, **cow**, **Kai**, **Kay**.

How?
By giving the child opportunities to hear, and see, you say short words that begin with **k** and to practise saying the words.

Resources
- At least three sets of the small pictures of short words that begin with **k** (p. 58).

Instructions
You are the speaker and the child is the listener in these activities.

1 Choose two pictures, e.g. **cow** and **key**. Put them on the table in front of the child and name them for her: '**Cow, Key.**' Tell the child to listen carefully and then you name one of the pictures placed in front of her, e.g. '**key**'. Then say 'What did I say?' The child listens and points to, or holds up, or puts a counter on the word she heard you say.

2 When you think the child is ready to listen and remember more words, choose three pictures, e.g. **cow, key** and **core**. Put them on the table in front of the child and name them for her: '**Cow. Key. Core.**' Tell the child to listen carefully and then you name two of the pictures placed in front of her, e.g. '**Cow. Core.**' Then say 'What did I say?' The child listens and points to, or holds up, or puts a counter on the words she heard you say. Increase the number of words to make the activity more challenging when you think the child is ready. For example, choose four pictures, name them, then name three of the four and ask the child to point to the three that you said.

Variations

- To make the activity more challenging, present at least three pictures to the child. Write down the words in the order you are going to say them, not in the order they appear in front of the child. For example, if the pictures in front of the child are **key**, **car**, **Kay**, you might write down **Kay**, **key**, **car**. Read out the words that you have written down: '**Kay**. **Key**. **Car**.' The child listens and arranges the pictures correspondingly, i.e. to match what you said (**Kay**, **key**, **car**). To do this activity, the child needs to be able to write, but not spell!

- Give the same pictures to yourself and to the child. You will need at least three, e.g. **car**, **key**, **cow**. Place a barrier between yourself and the child so that you cannot see each other's pictures. Arrange your pictures without the child seeing. Name the pictures in the order you have arranged them, e.g. '**Key**. **Car**. **Cow**.' The child listens and arranges her pictures to match what you have said. Remove the barrier and see if the child's pictures are in the same order as yours! Vary the activity by, for example, giving the child four pictures but only saying three of them. Reverse the game so that the child is the speaker and you are the listener.

Tips

Help! The child can't remember what I said! What can I do?

- Start this activity by asking the child to remember one picture. Show her two pictures, e.g. **cow** and **core**, and name one of the pictures, e.g. '**Core**'. The child listens and points to the one that she heard. If she can do this easily, make the activity more challenging by presenting the child with three pictures, e.g. **cow**, **core** and **key**, and naming two of them, e.g. '**Core**. **Key**.' Gradually increase the number of pictures so that the child has to remember more words. If she can't remember what you said, try reducing the number of pictures you are using, e.g. use three pictures instead of four.

Help! The child can't write the words! What can I do?

- To take part in this activity, children have to be able to read what they have written to you, but this does not mean that they have to spell the words correctly. For example, they might write **kee** for **key**. Ask an adult or another child to help.

- Draw pictures of the words you are going to say to the child, instead of writing the words. The child can draw pictures of the words she is going to say in the activity. She might need some help from an adult or another child.

Help! It's really hard work to get the child to do these activities! What can I do?

- Make sure you don't do these activities for too long. If the child finds it hard to concentrate, keep the activities short and fun!

- Offer a reward to the child if she does, say, one activity. Choose a reward that you know she will enjoy, e.g. blowing bubbles, playing with Lego for five minutes. Gradually increase the number of activities she has to do in order to get the reward!

Note: These tips can also help you work on the words in Sections 4, 5 and 6.

What's the word? (Listening activity)

Aim
To say short words that begin with the speech sound **k**: key, car, core, cow, Kai, Kay.

How?
By giving the child opportunities to hear, and see, you say short words that begin with **k** and to practise saying the words.

Resources
- At least three sets of the small pictures of short words that begin with **k** (p. 58).

Instructions
This activity is for children aged four and a half upwards.

1 Lay a set of the six small pictures in front of the child. Name them with the child: 'Car. Key. Core. Cow. Kai. Kay', so that she can hear the words before you start the activity.

2 Tell the child to listen carefully and point to the picture you are naming. Break words into the first speech sound, **k**, and the vowel, e.g. '**k – ar**' Leave a short pause between **k** and the vowel to help the child do this task. The child has to put the **k** and the vowel together in her head to make the word, **car**, and then point to the picture of a car.

3 When the child is familiar with this activity, ask her to put the sounds together in her head, e.g. **k – ar**, point to the picture and say the word out loud: '**car**'.

Variations
- Give one set of the small pictures to yourself and one to the child. Choose at least three pictures. Do not show the child the pictures you have chosen. Place a barrier between yourself and the child so that you cannot see each other's pictures.

- Arrange your pictures without the child seeing them on your side of the barrier, e.g. **Kay, cow, key**. Tell the child to listen carefully, find the pictures you say and put them on her side of the barrier. Break each word into the first sound, **k**, and the vowel, e.g. '**K – ay, k – ow, k – ey (k – ee)**.' The child has to put the **k** and the vowel together in her head, find the picture and put it behind her barrier. When you have finished, ask the child to say what the pictures are, e.g. '**Kay, cow, key**'. Remove the barrier to see if they are the same as your pictures.

Tips

Help! The child keeps pointing to the wrong pictures! What can I do?
- This activity might be very new for the child. Help her get used to it, and reduce any pressure she might be feeling, by using a toy or a puppet in the activity. Follow the instructions with the toy or puppet, so that the child can watch and listen. When the toy or puppet points to a picture, say 'Hold on a minute'. Turn to the child and say, for example: '**K** – **ar**. Let's put them together, **k** [pause] **ar**, **car**! Did the puppet point to the **car**? He did, didn't he? Clever puppet! He got it right!' When the child is more familiar with the activity, the puppet or toy can start to make some mistakes. For example: you say '**k** – **ore**' and the puppet points to the picture of a key.

- Check the puppet or toy's answer with the child and see if she can help the puppet by pointing to the right picture (core).

*Help! When the child blends **k** and **ar**, she says **gar** (or **tar**)! What can I do?*
- This is primarily a listening activity, not a speaking activity. If the child points to the right picture, e.g. **car**, then you know that she has blended **k** and **ar** together correctly in her head. The child said **gar** because she cannot say **k** in words yet.

- Say the word correctly for the child so that she has another opportunity to hear it and then ask her to repeat the word. For example: '**Car**. [child repeats] Good work! **K** – **ar**. **Car**! [child repeats] You got it!'

Note: These tips can also help you work on the words in Sections 4, 5 and 6.

What's the word? (Speaking activity)

Aim
To say short words that begin with the speech sound **k**: **key, car, core, cow, Kai, Kay**.

How?
By giving the child opportunities to hear, and see, you say short words that begin with **k** and to practise saying the words.

Resources

- A set of the small pictures (p. 58) that have shapes on the back (photocopy the sheet of shapes (p. 28) onto the back of the pictures).

- A dice

- The template for a dice with a different shape on each face (p. 30).

Instructions

1 Spread out the pictures in front of the child, face down so that you cannot see the pictures but you can see the shapes on the back.

2 Roll the dice with shapes on it. The shapes on the dice match the shapes on the back of the pictures. Turn over the picture that has the same shape as the dice, e.g. a circle, so that you can see what the picture is, e.g. **Kay**.

3 Roll the dice with numbers on it. You have to say the word on your picture, e.g. **Kay**, the number of times that you throw on the dice, e.g. five, '**Kay, Kay, Kay, Kay, Kay.**' Make sure you have the first turn so that you can demonstrate the activity to the child.

Variations

- Make the game competitive: the winner is the first person to say the names of all of the six pictures in the activity, i.e. to throw all of the shapes on the dice.

- Roll the dice with shapes on it and turn over the picture that has the same shape on it, e.g. a heart. Take it in turns to see how many times you can say the word in a minute. Use a one-minute salt timer.

My progress

Date	I can ...	☺/☹	I need to work on ...
	Listen carefully and hear short words that begin with **k**, e.g. **car**, **key**, **cow**, without any help.		
	Listen carefully and hear short words that begin with **k**, e.g. **car**, **key**, **cow**, with help.		
	Say **k** at the beginning of short words, e.g. **car**, **key**, **cow**, without any help.		
	Say **k** at the beginning of short words, e.g. **car**, **key**, **cow**, with some help.		

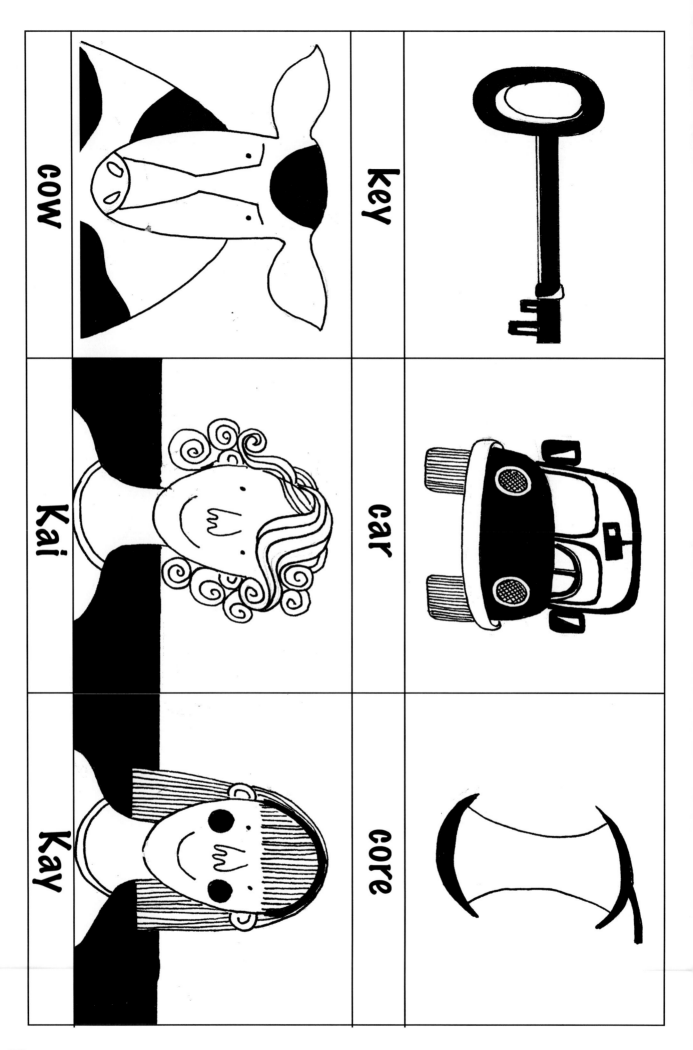

key

cow

car

Kai

core

Kay

Look!

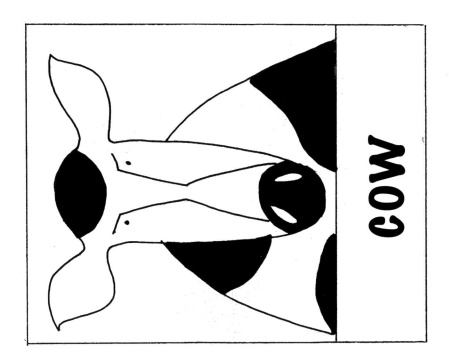

cow

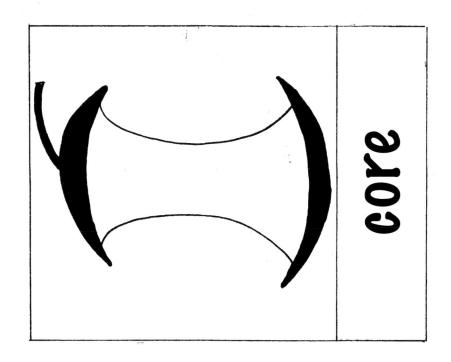

core

59

Look!

key

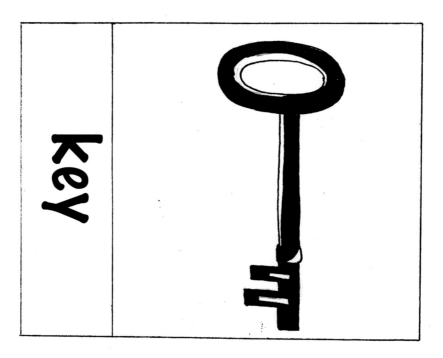

car

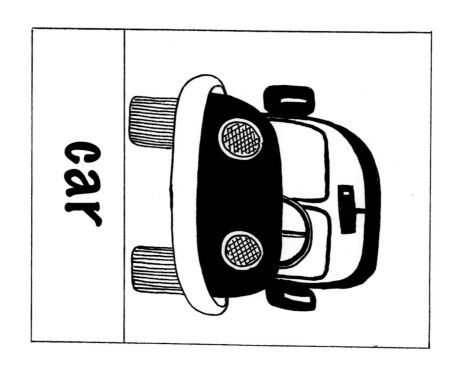

Look!

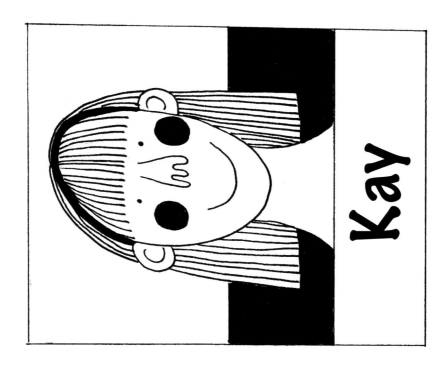

Kay

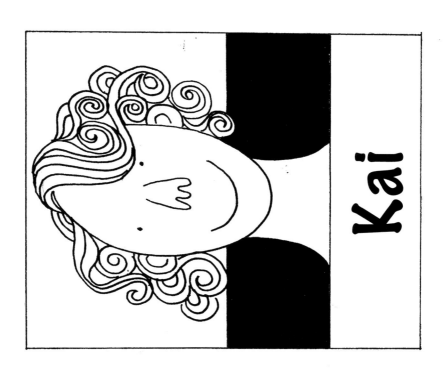

Kai

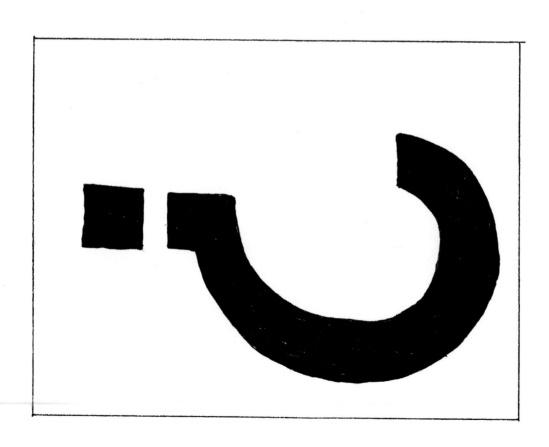

Close your eyes! I'm going to hide the cat!
Open your eyes! Where's the cat?

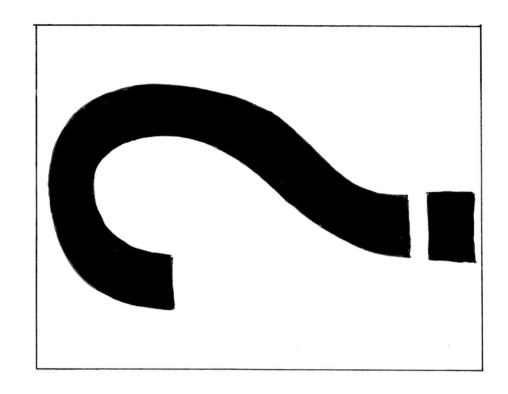

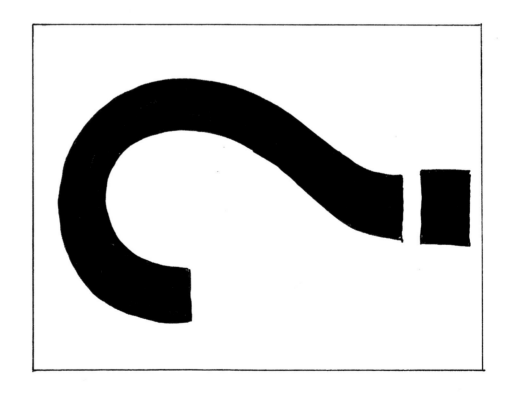

What's the next step?

- I can listen carefully and hear short words that begin with **k**, e.g. **car**, **key**, **cow**, without any help. **Play listening games from the list of games in Section 8, e.g. Listen and colour, Catch a picture, Bowling. Start Section 4.**

- I can listen carefully and hear short words that begin with **k**, e.g. **car**, **key**, **cow**, with help. **Continue playing listening games from Section 3. Play listening games from the list of games in Section 8. When the child is able to listen and hear short words that begin with k without help at least 70 per cent of the time, gradually introduce listening games from Section 4.**

- I can say **k** at the beginning of short words, e.g. **car**, **key**, **cow**, without any help. **Play speaking games from the list of games in Section 8, e.g. Pairs, Kim's game, Find the coin. Start Section 4.**

- I can say **k** at the beginning of short words, e.g. **car**, **key**, **cow**, with some help. **Continue playing talking games from Section 3 and carry on doing mouth exercises from Section 1. Play games from the list of games in Section 8. When the child is able to say k at the beginning of short words that begin with k without help at least 70 per cent of the time, gradually introduce speaking games from Section 4.**

Jingles

Many children, especially young children, e.g. under five, benefit from listening to words that contain the speech sound they are learning to use, in this case **k**. Listening can help raise their awareness of the speech sound in words such as **key**, and so help them to say the speech sound.

At the end of Sections 3, 4, 5 and 6 of this book there are some jingles that contain the words you have been working on with the child, for example in this section the short words that begin with **k**: **key**, **car**, **core**, **cow**, **Kai**, **Kay**.

Ideas for using the jingles

Step 1: Choose one or two jingles that contain the words you have been working on with the child.

Step 2: Read the jingle to the child and look at the pictures together. Read at least one jingle at the same time in each session, perhaps at the end. Some children may benefit from hearing the same jingle every day for a week, others may benefit from hearing one jingle for half the week and then hearing a new one for the rest of the week.

Tip

- Use your voice to make the jingles more interesting. For example, vary your pitch – say some words in a low voice, others in a high voice; vary your volume – say some words in a loud voice, others in a quiet voice. At this stage, there is no pressure on the child to talk. She can enjoy listening to the jingles without worrying about talking.

Step 3: When the child is making progress with the speech sound you are working on, for example she is saying **k** at the beginning of short words 70 per cent of the time, leave a word that contains **k** out in a line of the jingle and leave a pause to see if the child can say the missing word to complete the jingle. For example: 'Kay saw Kai in a _____ (car).' Gradually increase the number of lines in a jingle that you are doing this with. For example: 'Kay saw Kai in a _____ (car). Kai saw Kay on a _____ (cow).'

Tip

- If the child cannot remember the word, sound it out for her, e.g. '**c – ow**'. See if she can put the sounds together and say the word: '**cow**'.

Step 4: When the child can say the word you leave out 70 per cent of the time, try leaving out more than one word in lines to see if she can complete the jingles. For example: 'Cow! Have you seen _____ (Kay's) door _____ (key)?'

Step 5: When the child can say more than one word to complete sentences (step 4), see if she can remember an entire line of a jingle! Start with short lines! For example: 'Kay saw Kai in a _____ (car). (Kai saw Kay on a cow.)' Try taking it in turns to say a line each of short jingles!

Step 6: Try reading jingles with older children, e.g. six to seven years old.

Jingles with short words that begin with k

Jingle 1   (pictures on pp. 69 and 70)

Listen

Kay saw Kai

Kai saw Kay

Kay saw Kai in a car

Kai saw Kay on a cow

Say the word

Kay saw _____ (Kai)

Kai saw _____ (Kay)

Kay saw Kai in a _____ (car)

Kai saw Kay on a _____ (cow)

Jingle 2   (pictures on pp. 72 and 73)

Listen

Where's Kai's car key?

Where's Kay's door key?

Cow! Have you seen Kai's car key?

'Moo!' said the cow

Cow! Have you seen Kay's door key?

'Moo!' said the cow

I think that means no!

Say the word

Where's Kai's car _____ (key)?

Where's _____ (Kay's) door key?

Cow! Have you seen Kai's car _____ (key)?

'Moo!' said the _____ (cow)

Cow! Have you seen _____ (Kay's) door key?

'Moo!' said the _____ (cow)

I think that means no!

Jingle 3 (pictures on p. 71 and 73)

Listen

Boo bay bee

I've got a key

Bee bay bow

I've got a cow

Bow bay bar

I've got a car

Boo bay bow bar

Say the word

Boo bay bee

I've got a _____ (key)

Bee bay bow

I've got a _____ (cow)

Bow bay bar

I've got a _____ (car)

Boo bay bow bar

Jingle 4 (pictures on p. 74)

Listen

Nen nan nin

Put your core in the bin

Nee noo nar

Put your key in the car

Noo nar nay

Say hello to Kay

Nee noo nie

Say goodbye to Kai

Say the word

Nen nan nin

Put your _____ (core) in the bin

Nee noo nar

Put your key in the _____ (car)

Noo nar nay

Say hello to _____ (Kay)

Nee noo nie

Say goodbye to _____ (Kai)

Look!

Kay

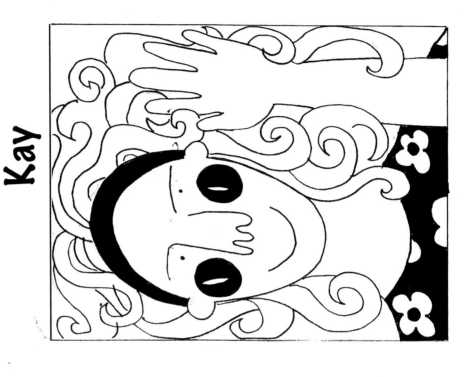

Kai

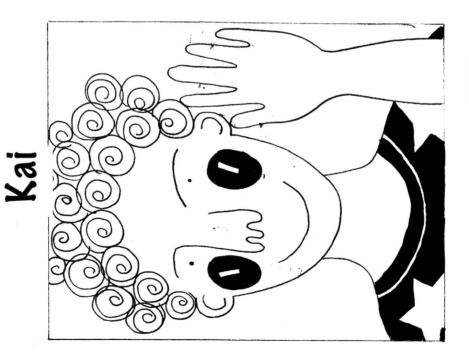

69

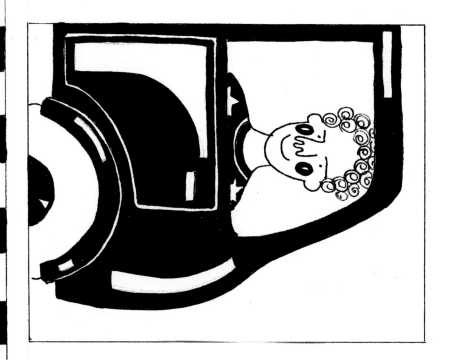

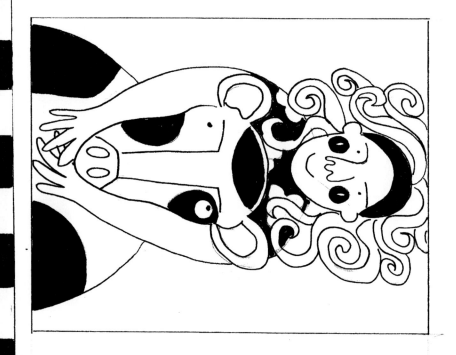

Look!

70

Look!

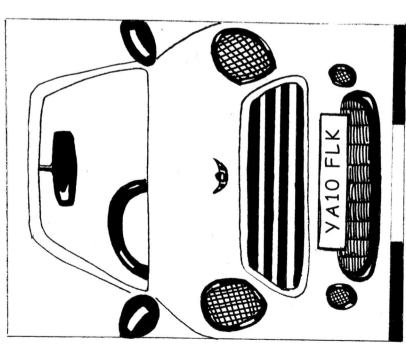

I've got a car

I've got a cow

Look!

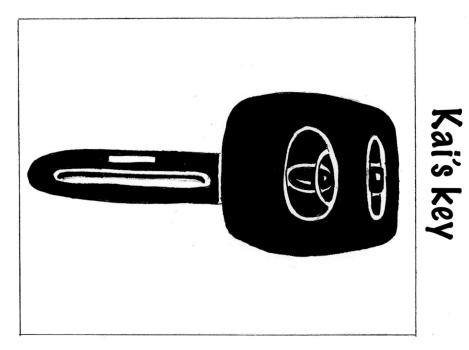

Kai's key

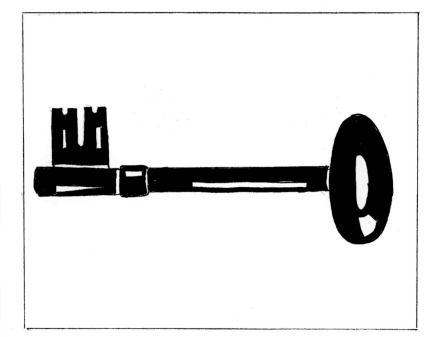

Kay's key

Look!

I've got a key

That means no!

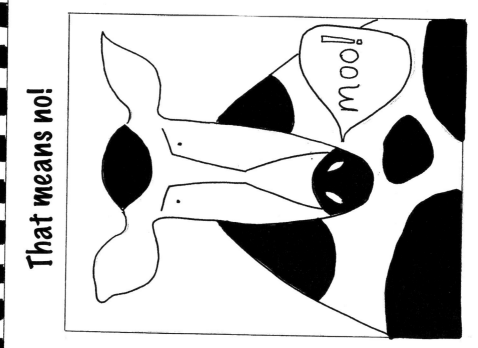

moo!

Look!

Put your key in the car

Put your core in the bin

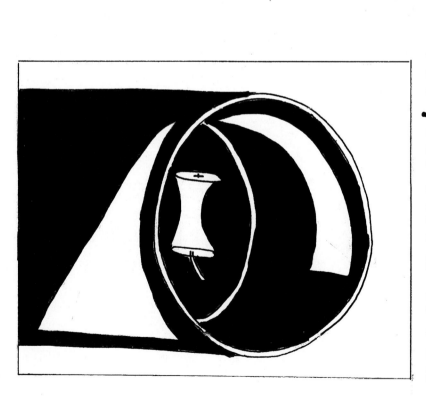

SECTION 4
SAYING K AT THE BEGINNING OF LONGER WORDS

Section 4: Saying k at the beginning of longer words

What's the picture? (Speaking activity)

Aim

To say longer words that begin with the speech sound **k**: **comb**, **corn**, **cup**, **cap**, **cat**, **kite**, **cake**, **cook**, **card**, **coat**, **Ken**, **Kate**, **coal**, **cork**, **can**, **curl**, **kiss**, **case**, **cot**, **cut**, **king**, **queen**.

How?

By giving the child opportunities to hear, and see, you say longer words that begin with **k** and to practise saying the words.

Resources

- Large pictures of longer words that begin with **k** (pp. 86–94).

- Small pictures of longer words that begin with **k** (pp. 95–98).

- Page of two doors with question marks on each one and the instruction *What's the picture?* (p. 64). You will need to photocopy this page and cut along three sides of the doors so that you can open them to reveal a picture.

Instructions

1 Put the page with the doors on top of large pictures of words that begin with **k**, e.g. **comb** and **kite**.

2 Read the instruction at the top of the page to the child: *What's the picture? Open the door and see!* Before you open the door to see what the picture is, say: 'My turn!' so that the child knows you are going first. Open the first door to reveal the picture and name it, e.g. 'Look! **Comb**!' so that the child has an opportunity to hear you say **k** at the beginning of a short word.

3 When you have finished your go, say to the child: 'Your turn!' so that he knows that it is his go to open the door and name the picture behind it.

4 Put the picture of the doors over different large pictures, e.g. **cork** and **curl**, and take it in turns to open a door and name the picture behind it. Follow this procedure to name all the large pictures on the pages for this activity.

Variation

- Tell the child to close his eyes and put a small picture of a word beginning with **k** behind each door. Then ask the child to open his eyes and open the doors. Try asking him to guess what picture is behind the door before he opens it.

Roll and say (Speaking activity)

Aim

To say longer words that begin with the speech sound **k**: **comb**, **corn**, **cup**, **cap**, **cat**, **kite**, **cake**, **cook**, **card**, **coat**, **Ken**, **Kate**, **coal**, **cork**, **can**, **curl**, **kiss**, **case**, **cot**, **cut**.

How?

By giving the child opportunities to hear, and see, you say longer words that begin with **k** and to practise saying the words.

Resources

- A set of the small pictures (pp. 95 – 98) that have shapes on the back (photocopy the sheet of shapes (p. 28) onto the back of the pictures).

- A dice

- The template for a dice with a different shape on each face (p. 30).

Instructions

1 Spread out the pictures in front of the child, face down, so that you cannot see them but you can see the shapes on the back.

2 Roll the dice with shapes on it. The shapes on the dice match the shapes on the back of the pictures. Turn over the picture that has the same shape as the dice, e.g. a circle, so that you can see what the picture is, e.g. **can**.

3 Roll the dice with numbers on it. You have to say the word on your picture, e.g. **can**, the number of times that you throw on the dice, e.g. five, '**can, can, can, can, can**.' Make sure you have the first turn so that you can demonstrate the activity to the child.

Variations

- Make the game competitive: the winner is the first person to say the names of all of the six pictures in the activity, i.e. to throw all of the shapes on the dice.

- Roll the dice with shapes on it and turn over the picture that has the same shape on it, e.g. a heart. Take it in turns to see how many times you can say the word in a minute. Use a one-minute salt timer.

Remember and say (Speaking and listening game)

Aim

To say longer words that begin with the speech sound **k**: **comb**, **corn**, **cup**, **cap**, **cat**, **kite**, **cake**, **cook**, **card**, **coat**, **Ken**, **Kate**, **coal**, **cork**, **can**, **curl**, **kiss**, **case**, **cot**, **cut**.

How?

By giving the child opportunities to hear, and see, you say words that begin with **k** and to practise saying the words.

Resources

- At least one set of the small pictures of words that begin with **k** (pp. 95 – 98),

Instructions

1 Look at the pictures of the longer words that begin with **k** and name them with the child.

2 Present at least two of the small pictures to the child and name them, e.g. '**Cup**. **Card**.' Tell the child to 'take a photo' of the pictures in his mind, i.e. use a mental camera, to help him remember them. Give him at least 30 seconds to look at the pictures. Then turn the pictures over and ask the child if he can remember what they are. The child then names the pictures. Turn them over to see if he is right.

   Make this activity more challenging by increasing the number of pictures that the child has to remember.

Variations

- Give the same pictures to yourself and to the child. You will need at least four, e.g. **cake**, **corn**, **coal**, **can**.

- Place a barrier between yourself and the child so that you cannot see each other's pictures. Arrange at least two of your pictures behind the barrier so that the child cannot see what they are. Name the pictures, e.g. '**Corn**. **Can**.'

- Pause for a few seconds and then say: 'Ready. Steady. Go!' The child listens, then looks at his pictures, finds the ones he heard you name and lays them out on his side of the barrier. When you remove the barrier, you will see if the child's pictures are the same as yours! Reverse the game so that the child names pictures for you to remember and arrange behind the barrier.

- Play *Kim's game* with the small pictures (see the instructions in Section 8, p.189).

- Play *Pairs* (see the instructions in Section 8, p.185).

Listen and guess (Listening and speaking activity)

Aim

To say longer words that begin with the speech sound **k**: **comb**, **corn**, **cup**, **cap**, **cat**, **kite**, **cake**, **cook**, **card**, **coat**, **Ken**, **Kate**, **coal**, **cork**, **can**, **curl**, **kiss**, **case**.

How

By giving the child opportunities to hear, and see, you say words that begin with **k** and to practise saying the words.

Resources

* A set of small pictures of longer words that begin with **k** (pp. 95 – 98).

Instructions

1   Choose a picture, e.g. **cap**. Do not show it to the child. Place it face down in front of him.

2   Tell the child at least three things about the picture, e.g. 'You wear it. You wear it on your head. It keeps the sun out of your eyes.'

3   The child guesses what the picture is and turns it over to see if he is right. Reverse the game so that the child chooses a picture and describes it and you guess what it is.

Variation

* To make this activity more challenging for the child, put at least three pictures in front of him, e.g. **cork**, **kite**, **card**.

* Choose one of the pictures to describe, e.g. **kite**. Do not tell the child which picture you have chosen. Tell him three things about the picture, e.g. 'You can fly this. It has a string that you hold on to. You can get big ones and little ones in any colour.' The child listens and points to the picture that he thinks you are describing, e.g. **kite**.

* To make this activity more challenging, choose at least three pictures. Do not show them to the child. Place them face down in front of him. Tell the child at least three things about the first picture. The child guesses what it is and turns it over to see if he is right or not. Then tell him three things about the second picture. The child guesses and checks if he is right or not. Follow the same procedure for the third picture. Reverse the game, so that the child chooses at least three pictures and describes them to you.

* Place a barrier between you and the child. Make sure that you and the child each have a set of the small pictures.

- Choose at least three pictures from your set, e.g. **coal**, **comb**, **case**. Describe the pictures to the child, leaving a pause between each description so that he can find the picture he thinks you are talking about in his set. When the child has found the picture he thinks you are describing, he puts it face up behind the barrier so that you cannot see it. When you have described all three pictures and the child has put three corresponding pictures behind the barrier, ask him to say what his pictures are, e.g. '**coal**, **comb**, **case**'. Then remove the barrier to see if he has the same pictures as you. Reverse the game, so that the child chooses and describes his pictures and you listen and try to find the corresponding picture in your set.

What did I say? (Listening and speaking activity)

Aim
To say longer words that begin with the speech sound **k**: **comb**, **corn**, **cup**, **cap**, **cat**, **kite**, **cake**, **cook**, **card**, **coat**, **Ken**, **Kate**, **coal**, **cork**, **can**, **curl**, **kiss**, **case**, **cot**, **cut**.

How?
By giving the child opportunities to hear, and see, you say longer words that begin with **k** and to practise saying the words.

Resources
- At least two sets of the small pictures of longer words that begin with **k** (pp. 95 – 98).

Instructions
You are the speaker and the child is the listener in these activities.

1 Choose two pictures, e.g. **case** and **coat**. Put them on the table in front of the child and name them for him, e.g. '**Case. Coat.**' Tell the child to listen carefully and then you name one of the pictures placed in front of him, e.g. '**Coat.**' Then say 'What did I say?' The child listens and points to, or holds up, or puts a counter on the picture of the word he heard you say.

2 When you think the child is ready to listen and remember more words, choose three pictures, e.g. **case**, **coat** and **coal**. Put them on the table in front of the child and name them for him, e.g. '**Case. Coat. Coal.**' Tell the child to listen carefully and then you name two of the pictures placed in front of him, e.g. '**Case. Coal.**' Then say 'What did I say?' The child listens and points to, or holds up, or puts a counter on the words he heard you say. Increase the number of words to make the activity more challenging when you think the child is ready. For example, choose four pictures, name them, then name three of the four and ask the child to point to the three that you said.

Variations

- To make the activity more challenging, present at least three pictures to the child. Write down the words in the order you are going to say them, not in the order they are in front of the child. For example, if the pictures in front of the child are **case**, **coal**, **coat**, you might write down **coal**, **case**, **coat**. Read out the words that you have written down: '**Coal**. **Case**. **Coat**.' The child listens and arranges the pictures correspondingly, i.e. to match what you said (**coal**, **case**, **coat**).

- To do this activity, the child needs to be able to write, but not spell!

- Give the same pictures to yourself and to the child. You will need at least three, e.g. **Kate**, **curl**, **kiss**. Place a barrier between yourself and the child so that you cannot see each other's pictures. Arrange your pictures without the child seeing. Name the pictures in the order you have arranged them, e.g. '**Curl**. **Kate**. **Kiss**.' The child listens and arranges his pictures to match what you have said. Remove the barrier and see if the child's pictures are in the same order as yours! Reverse the game so that the child is the speaker and you are the listener.

What's the word? (Listening activity)

Aim

To say longer words that begin with the speech sound **k**: **comb**, **corn**, **cup**, **cap**, **cat**, **kite**, **cake**, **cook**, **card**, **coat**, **Ken**, **Kate**, **coal**, **cork**, **can**, **curl**, **kiss**, **case**, **cot**, **cut**, **king**, **queen**.

How?

By giving the child opportunities to hear, and see, you say longer words that begin with **k** and to practise saying the words.

Resources

- At least two sets of the small pictures of longer words that begin with **k** (pp. 95 – 98).

Instructions

This activity is for children aged four and a half upwards.

1. Place a set of the small pictures in front of the child. Name them with the child: '**Comb**. **Corn**. **Cup**. **Cap**. **Cat**. **Kite**. **Cake**. **Cook**. **Card**. **Coat**. **Ken**. **Kate**. **Cork**. **Coal**. **Can**. **Curl**. **Kiss**. **Case**. **Cut**. **Cot**', so that he can hear the words before you start the activity.

Use at least three small pictures with younger children. Be flexible with the number of pictures you present at the beginning of the activity, depending on the level of the child.

Avoid using pictures of words that contain speech sounds the child cannot yet say in speaking activities. For example, most children usually start using the speech sounds **s** in their talking at between two and a half and three years of age and the speech sound **l** between the age of three and three and a half (Grunwell, 1987). Although children usually start using the speech sound **t** between one and a half and two years of age, some children say noisy speech sounds instead of quiet speech sounds, e.g. **d** instead of **t**, **b** instead of **p**.

2   Tell the child to listen carefully and point to the picture you are naming. Break words into the first speech sound, **k**, and the rest of the word, e.g. '**c – an**'. Leave a short pause between the speech sounds to help the child carry out this task.

The child has to put the speech sounds together in his head, e.g. **can**, and point to the picture of a can.

3   When the child is familiar with this activity, ask him to put the sounds together in his head, e.g. **c – an**, point to the picture and say the word out loud, e.g. '**can**'.

Variations

• Give one set of the small pictures to yourself and one to the child. Choose at least three. Do not show the child the pictures you have chosen. Place a barrier between yourself and the child so that you cannot see each other's pictures.

• Arrange your pictures without the child seeing them on your side of the barrier, e.g. **Ken**, **cup**, **kite**. Tell the child to listen carefully, find the pictures you say and put them on his side of the barrier. Break each word into the first sound, **k**, and the rest of the word, e.g. '**K – en**, **c – up**, **k – ite**.' The child has to put the speech sounds together in his head, find the picture and put it behind his barrier. When you have finished, ask the child to say what the pictures are, e.g. '**Ken. Cup. Kite.**' Remove the barrier to see if they are the same as your pictures.

• Challenge older children by breaking words into three parts, e.g. '**K – e – n, c – u – p**.'

Tips

Help! The child keeps pointing to the wrong pictures! What can I do?

- This activity might be very new for the child. Help him get used to it, and reduce any pressure he might be feeling, by using a toy or a puppet. Follow the instructions with the toy or puppet, so that the child can watch and listen. When the toy or puppet points to a picture, say, for example: 'Hold on a minute.' Turn to the child and say, for example: '**C** – **up**. Let's put them together. **C** – **up**. **Cup**! Did he point to the **cup**? He did, didn't he? Clever puppet! He got it right!' When the child is more familiar with the activity, the puppet or toy can start to make some mistakes. For example: you say '**c** – **an**' and the puppet or toy points to the picture of a comb. Check the puppet or toy's answer with the child and see if the child can help the puppet or toy by pointing to the right picture.

*Help! When the child tries to say longer words that begin with **k**, e.g. **cap**, he says **t**! He says **tap** instead of **cap**! What can I do?*

- This is primarily a listening activity, not a speaking activity. If the child points to the right picture, e.g. **cap**, you know that he has blended **c** and **ap** together correctly in his head. The child said **tap** because he cannot say **k** in words yet. Say the word correctly for the child so that he has another opportunity to hear it. For example: '**Cap**. [child repeats] Good work! **C** – **ap**. **Cap**! [child repeats] You got it!'

*How can I help the child to say the speech sound **k** in words?*

- You will need two coins or Lego bricks and small pictures of the words that you are working on with the child, e.g. **comb**, **cap**, **can**, **coal**. Choose one of the pictures, e.g. **cap**. Put the two coins or Lego bricks in front of the child, leaving a gap between the two objects. Touch the first coin or brick and say the first sound of the word: **k**. Then touch the second coin or brick and say the rest of the word, e.g. **ap** (**cap**). Take it in turns to touch the coins or bricks and say **k** and **ap** as you touch each one. Gradually move the two objects closer together so that the pause you leave between saying **k** and saying **ap** is smaller and smaller, until the coins or bricks are touching and there is no gap between **k** and **ap**, i.e. you are saying **kap** (**cap**).

- Instead of asking the child to say **k** – **ap**, try asking him to say **ka**, leave a pause and then say **p** (**ka** – **p**). Saying a speech sound and doing a movement, e.g. touching a brick, touching one of your fingers, jumping on a mat, helps some children to say words. Use coins or bricks as described in the previous tip. Or try putting two mats or pieces of paper or paper footprints on the floor for the child to step or jump on when he says **ka** and **p**. Or try putting paper hands on a wall for the child to touch when he says **ka** and **p**. Gradually bring the two mats or pieces of paper together until they are touching and there is no gap between **ka** and **p**, i.e. you are saying **kap** (**cap**).

My progress

Date	I can ...	☺/☹	I need to work on ...
	Listen carefully and hear words that begin with **k**, e.g. **can**, **cap**, **comb**, without any help.		
	Listen carefully and hear words that begin with **k**, e.g. **can**, **cap**, **comb**, with help.		
	Say **k** at the beginning of words, e.g. **can**, **cap**, **comb**, without any help.		
	Say **k** at the beginning of words, e.g. **can**, **cap**, **comb**, with some help.		

cut

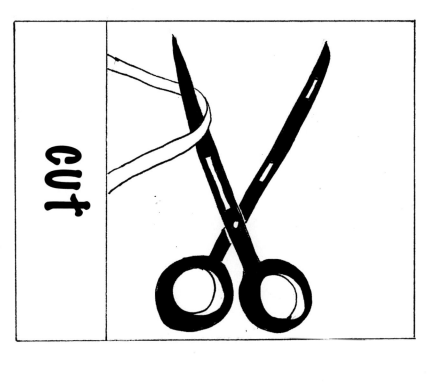

cot

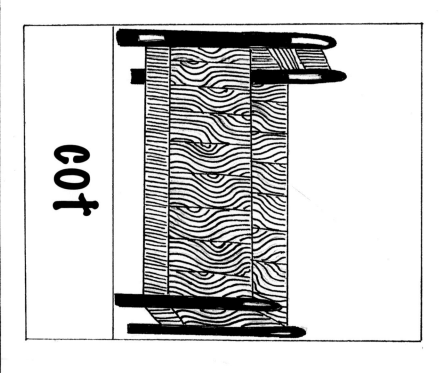

Look!

Look!

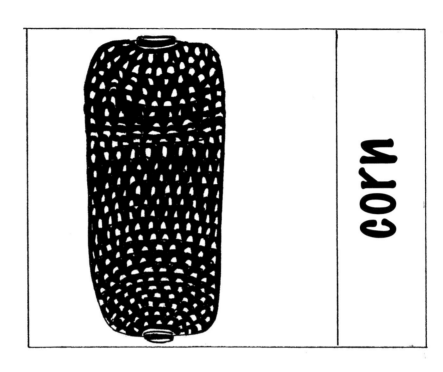

corn

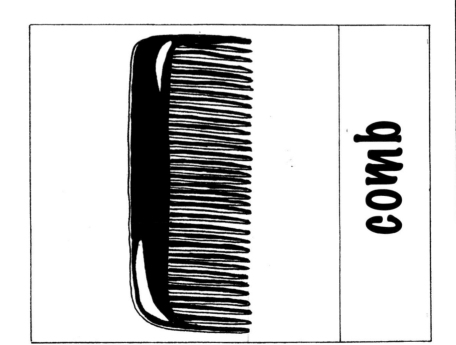

comb

Look!

cat

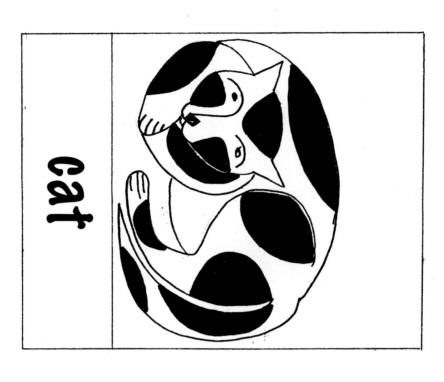

kite

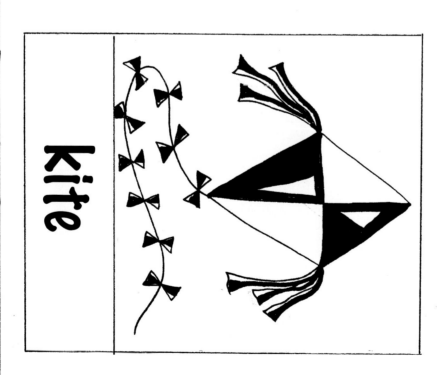

Look!

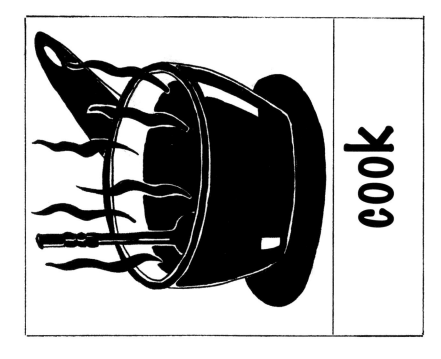

cook

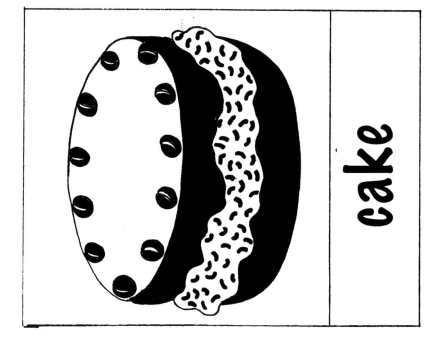

cake

coat

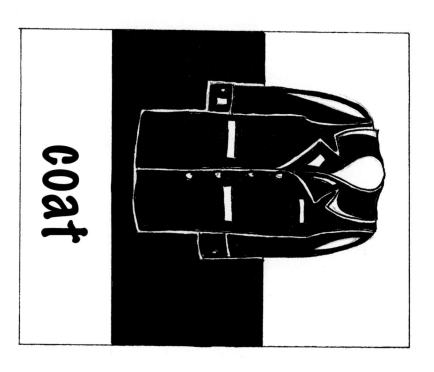

card

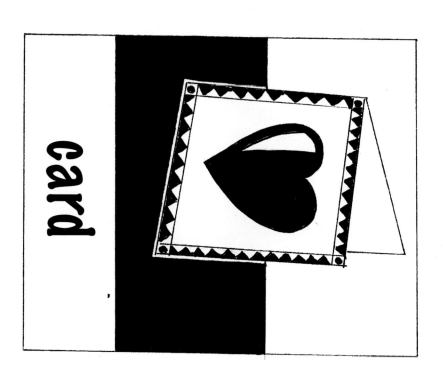

Look!

Look!

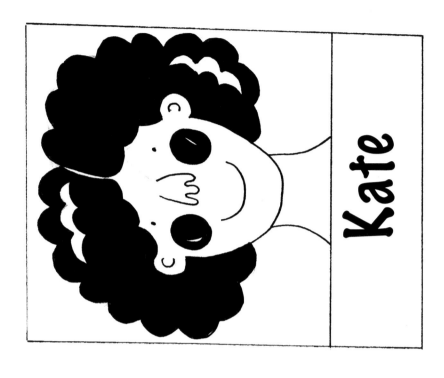

Kate

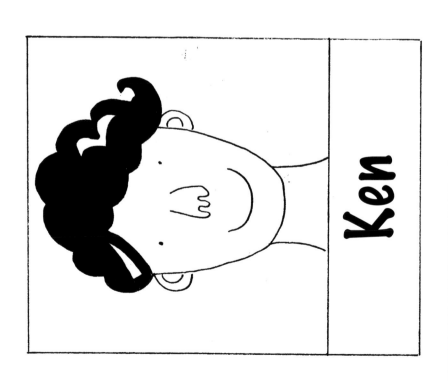

Ken

Look!

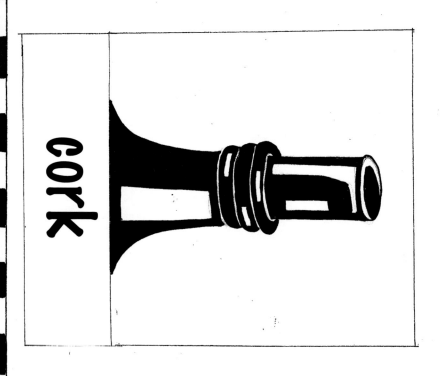

cork

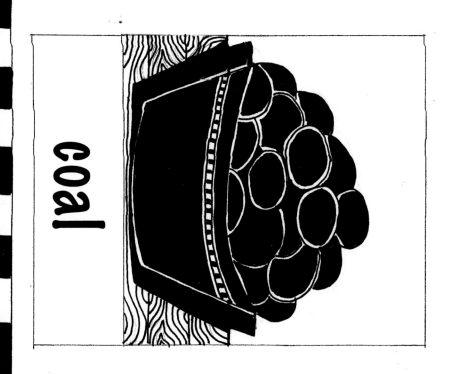

coal

Look!

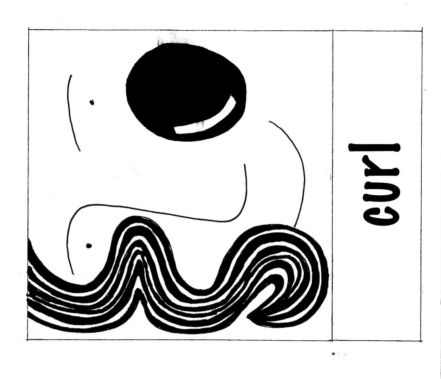

curl

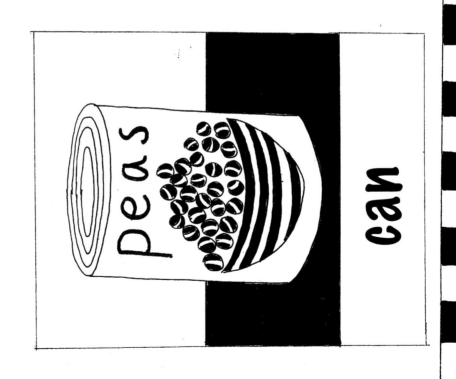

can

Look!

case

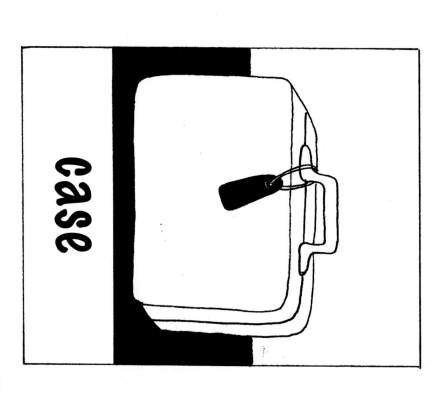

kiss

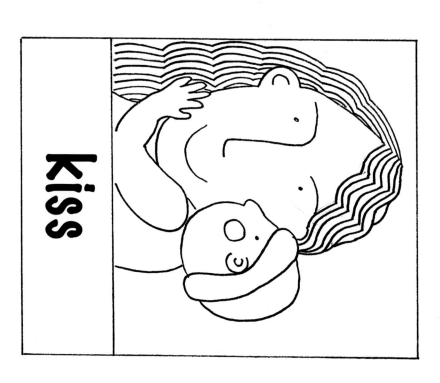

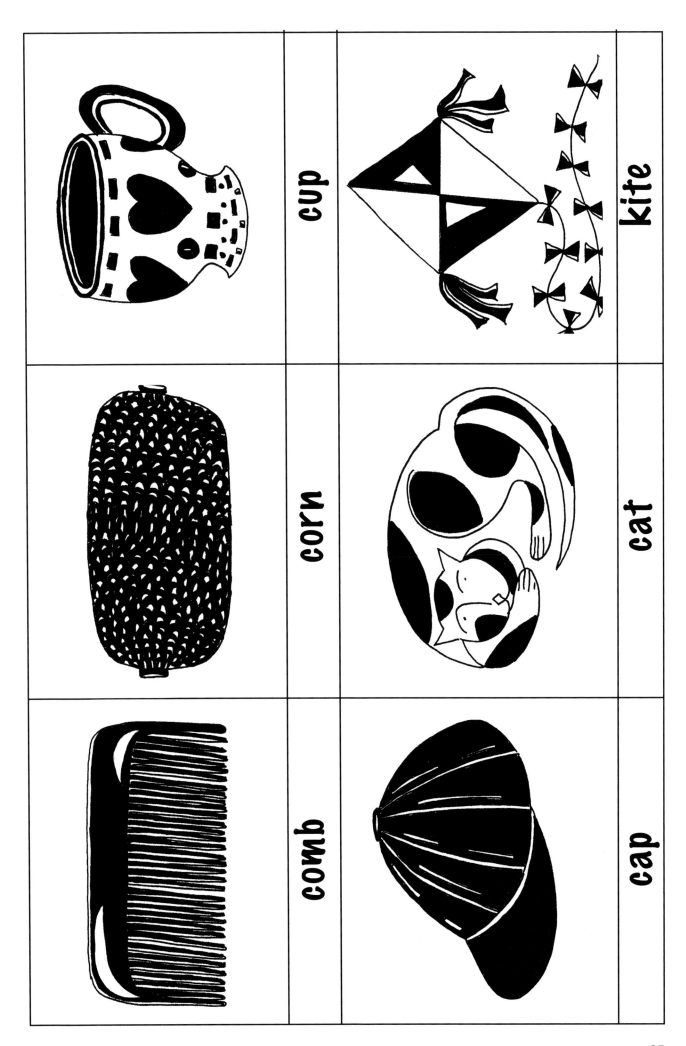

cup

kite

corn

cat

comb

cap

95

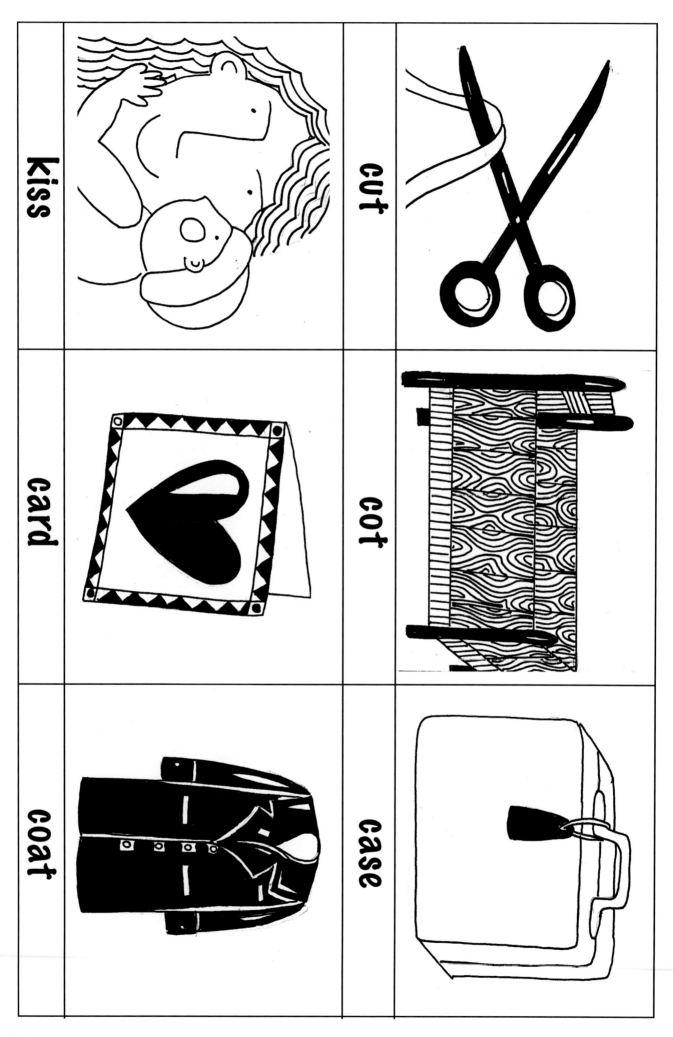

cut

kiss

cot

card

case

coat

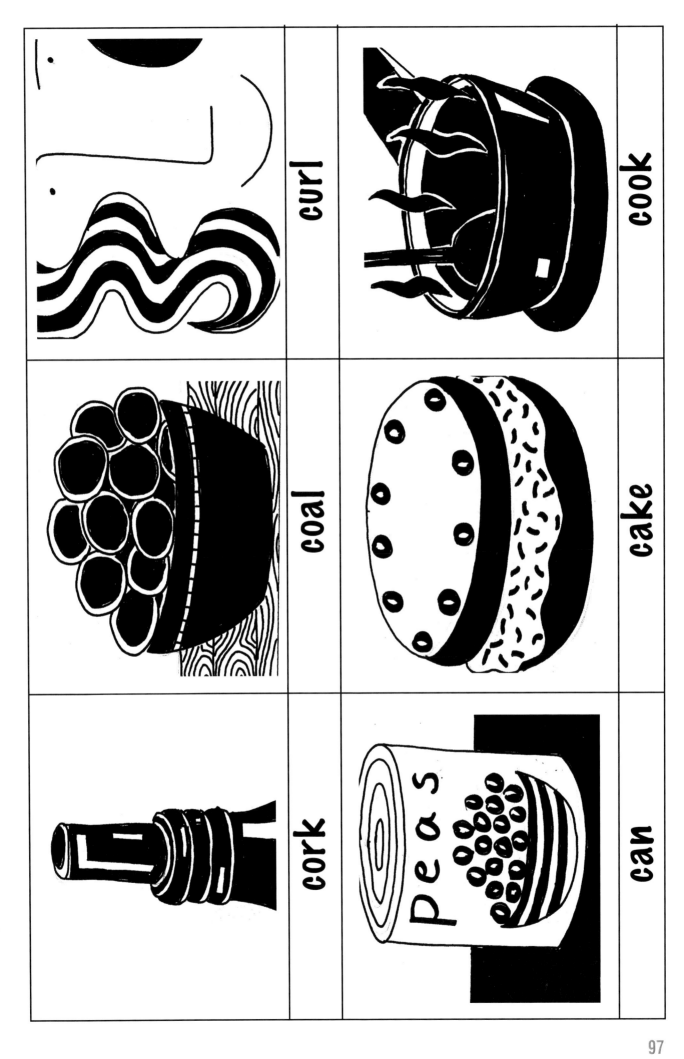

curl

cook

coal

cake

cork

can

Ken

Kate

What's the next step?

- I can listen carefully and hear words that begin with **k**, e.g. **can**, **cap**, **comb**, without any help. **Start doing listening activities in Section 5. Play listening games from the list of games in Section 8, e.g. Goal!, Listen and colour.**

- I can listen carefully and hear words that begin with **k**, e.g. **can**, **cap**, **comb**, with help. **Carry on doing listening activities in Section 4. Use games from Section 2 and play listening games from the list of games in Section 8, e.g. Bowling, Catch a picture. Start introducing listening activities from Section 5 when the child can hear words that begin with k in activities at least 70 per cent of the time.**

- I can say **k** at the beginning of words, e.g. **can**, **cap**, **comb**, without any help. **Start working on Section 5. Play speaking games from the list of games in Section 8, e.g. Guess what?, What is it?**

- I can say **k** at the beginning of words, e.g. **can**, **cap**, **comb**, with some help. **Carry on playing talking games from Section 4 and carry on doing mouth exercises from Section 1. Play games from the list of games in Section 8. When the child is able to say k at the beginning of longer words that begin with k without help at least 70 per cent of the time, gradually introduce speaking games from Section 5.**

Jingles with words that begin with k

See the advice at the end of Section 3 on how to use the jingles in sessions (pp. 64 – 65).

Jingle 1 (picture on p. 103)

Listen

Rock a bye baby,

Cat's in the cot!

Kiss it goodnight

And turn out the light

Night, night cat

Sleep well!

Say the word

Rock a bye baby,

Cat's in the _____ (cot)!

_____ (Kiss) it goodnight

And turn out the light

Night, night _____ (cat)

Sleep well!

Jingle 2 (pictures on p. 104)

Listen

Look at the king's hair! Where's his comb?

He needs a hair cut!

Quick! Comb his hair!

'Ow!' said the king, 'Ow!'

Poor king! Give him some cake!

Cake and a cup of tea!

'Yum!' said the king

Say the word

Look at the king's hair! Where's his_____ (comb)?

He needs a hair _____ (cut)!

Quick! _____ (Comb) his hair!

'Ow!' said the _____ (king), 'Ow!'

Poor king! Give him some _____ (cake)!

Cake and a _____ (cup) of tea!

'Yum!' said the _____ (king)

Jingle 3   (pictures on p. 105)

Listen

Look! A cat in a coat!

Look! A cat carrying a case!

Look! A cat in a cap!

Look! A cat flying a kite!

Look! A cat eating a cake!

What a clever cat!

Say the word

Look! A cat in a _____ (coat)!

Look! A cat carrying a _____ (case)!

Look! A cat in a _____ (cap)!

Look! A cat flying a _____ (kite)!

Look! A cat eating a _____ (cake)!

What a clever _____ (cat)!

Jingle 4   (pictures on p. 106)

Listen

The king can cook. He can cook yummy cakes!

The queen can't cook. She makes yukky cakes!

The queen can drive a car.

The king can't drive a car, but he can ride a bike.

Can you ride a bike?

Say the word

The king can _____ (cook). He can cook yummy _____ (cakes)!

The queen can't_____ (cook). She makes yukky ____ (cakes)!

The queen can drive a _____ (car).

The king can't drive a _____ (car) but he can ride a bike.

Can you ride a bike?

Jingle 5 (pictures on p. 107)

Listen

Can you cook a kite?

No. I can't!

Can you fly a cot?

No. I can't!

Can you sleep in a cup?

No. I can't!

Can you drink a cake?

No. I can't!

But I can cook a cake, I can fly a kite, I can sleep in a cot and I can drink tea in a cup.

Say the word

Can you cook a _____ (kite)?

No. I _____ (can't)!

Can you fly a _____ (cot)?

No. I _____ (can't)!

Can you sleep in a _____ (cup)?

No. I _____ (can't)!

Can you drink a _____ (cake)?

No. I _____ (can't)!

But I can cook a _____ (cake), I can fly a _____ (kite), I can sleep in a _____ (cot) and I can drink tea in a _____ (cup).

Night, night cat!

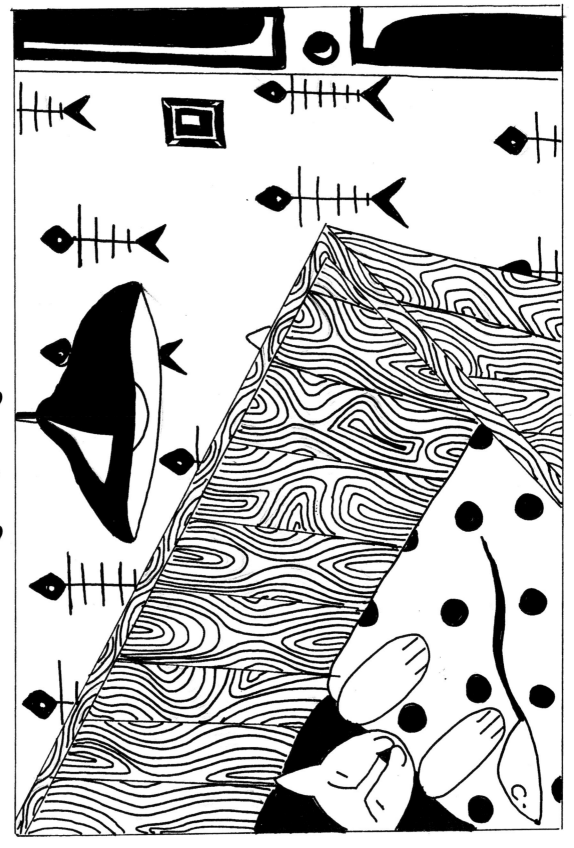

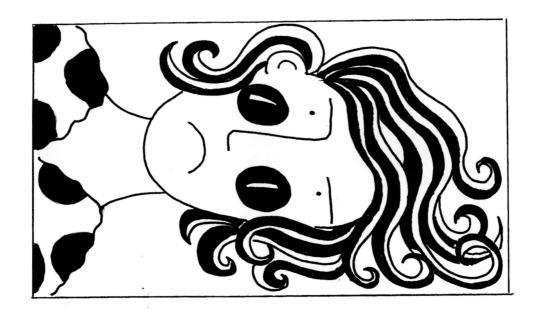

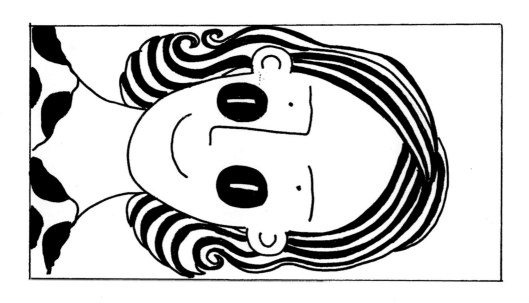

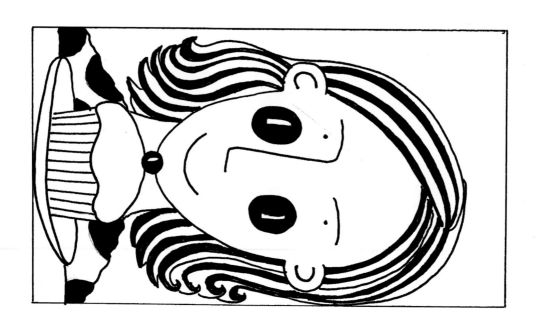

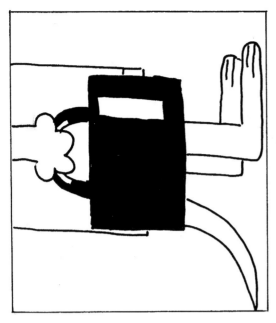
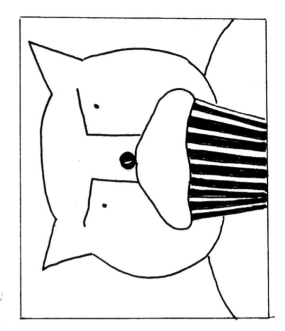
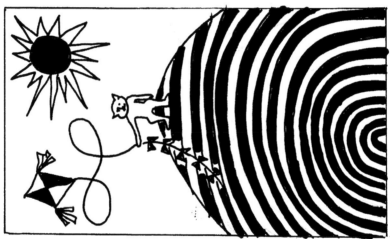
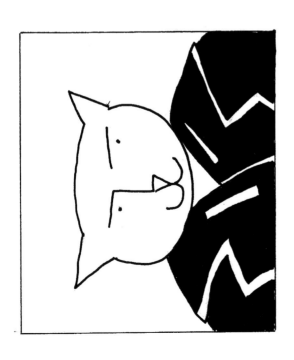
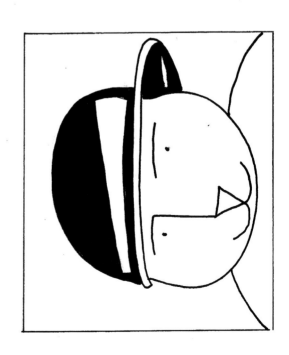

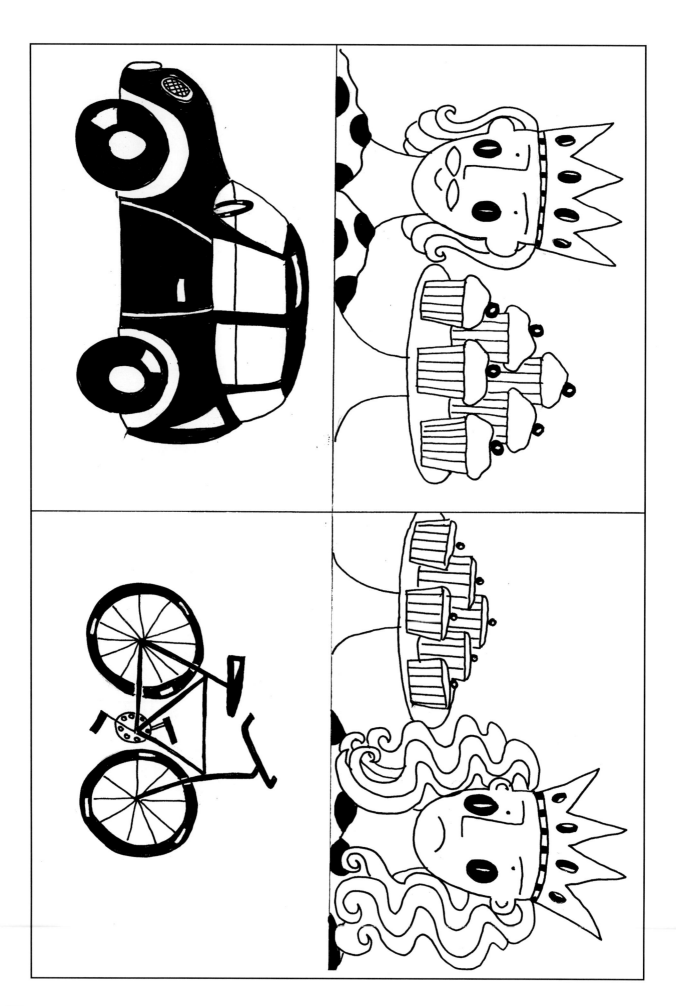

Fly a cot!

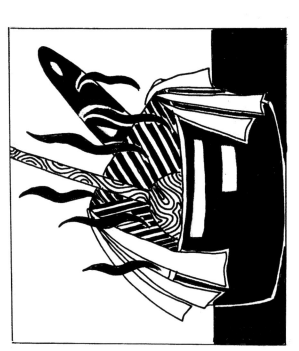

Cook a kite!

Drink a cake!

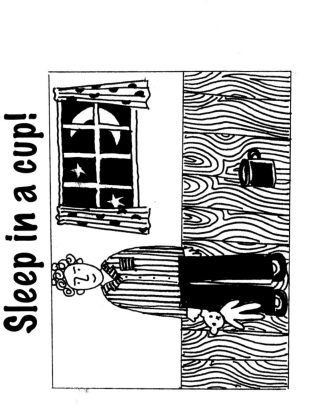

Sleep in a cup!

SECTION 5

SAYING K AT THE END OF LONGER WORDS

Section 5: **Saying k at the end of longer words**

What's the picture? (Speaking activity)

Aim
To say longer words that end with the speech sound **k: book, duck, sack, lake, beak, bike, fork, sock, shark, Mark, dark, back, lock, park**.

How?
By giving the child opportunities to hear, and see, you say longer words that end with **k** and to practise saying the words.

Resources
- Large pictures of longer words that end with **k** (pp. 122–128).

- Small pictures of longer words that end with **k** (pp. 119–121).

- Page of two doors with question marks on each one and the instruction *What's the picture?* (p. 62). You will need to photocopy this page and cut along three sides of the doors so that you can open them to reveal a picture.

Instructions
1 Put the page with the doors on top of large pictures of words that end with **k**, e.g. **duck** and **fork**.

2 Read the instruction at the top of the page to the child: *What's the picture? Open the door and see!*. Before you open the door to see what the picture is, say: 'My turn!' so that the child knows you are going first. Open the first door to reveal the picture and name it, e.g. 'Look! **Duck**!' so that the child has an opportunity to hear you say **k** at the end of a longer word.

3 When you have finished your go, say to the child: 'Your turn!' so that she knows that it is her go to open the door and name the picture behind it.

4 Put the picture of the doors over different large pictures, e.g. **shark** and **lock**, and take it in turns to open a door and name the picture behind it. Follow this procedure to name all the large pictures on pages 122–128.

Variation
- Tell the child to close her eyes and put a small picture of a word ending with **k** behind each door. Then ask the child to open her eyes and open the doors. Try asking her to guess which picture is behind the door before she opens it.

Roll and say (Speaking activity)

Aim

To say longer words that end with the speech sound **k**: **book**, **duck**, **sack**, **lake**, **beak**, **bike**, **fork**, **sock**, **shark**, **Mark**, **dark**, **back**, **lock**, **park**.

How?

By giving the child opportunities to hear, and see, you say words that end with **k** and to practise saying the words.

Resources

- A set of the small pictures (pp.119–121) with shapes on the back (photocopy the sheet of shapes (p. 28) onto the back of the pictures).

- A dice

- The template for a dice with a different shape on each face (p. 30).

Instructions

1 Spread the pictures out in front of the child, face down, so that you cannot see the pictures but you can see the shapes on the back.

2 Roll the dice with shapes on it. The shapes on the dice match the shapes on the back of the pictures. Turn over the picture that has the same shape as the dice, e.g. circle, so that you can see what the picture is, e.g. **book**.

3 Roll the dice with numbers on it. You have to say the word on your picture, e.g. **book**, the number of times that you throw on the dice, e.g. five, '**book, book, book, book, book**.' Make sure you have the first turn so that you can demonstrate the activity to the child.

Variations

- Make the game competitive: the winner is the first person to say the names of all of the six pictures in the activity, i.e. to throw all of the shapes on the dice.

- Roll the dice with shapes on it and turn over the picture that has the same shape on it, e.g. a heart. Take it in turns to see how many times you can say the word in a minute. Use a one-minute salt timer.

Remember and say (Listening and speaking activity)

Aim

To say longer words that end with the speech sound **k**: **book**, **duck**, **sack**, **lake**, **beak**, **bike**, **fork**, **sock**, **shark**, **Mark**, **dark**, **back**, **lock**, **park**.

How?

By giving the child opportunities to hear, and see, you say words that end with **k** and to practise saying the words.

Resources

- At least one set of the small pictures of words that end with **k** (pp.119–121).

Instructions

1   Look at the pictures of the words that end with **k** and name them with the child (see the tips below on choosing which pictures to present to which children).

Tips

- Use at least three small pictures with younger children. Be flexible with the number of pictures you use at the beginning of the activity, depending on the level of the child.

- Avoid using pictures of words that contain speech sounds the child cannot yet say in speaking activities. For example, most children usually start using the speech sounds **s** and **f** in their talking at between two and a half and three years of age, the speech sound **l** between the age of three and three and a half, and **sh** between three and a half and four years of age (Grunwell, 1987).

2   Present at least two of the pictures to the child and name them, e.g. '**Bike**. **Mark**.' Tell the child to 'take a photo' of the pictures in her mind, i.e. use a mental camera, to help her remember them. Give her at least 30 seconds to look at the pictures. Then turn the pictures over and ask the child if she can remember what they are. The child then names the pictures. Turn them over to see if she is right. Make this activity more challenging by increasing the number of pictures that the child has to remember.

Variations

- Give the same pictures to yourself and to the child. You will need at least four, e.g. **book**, **fork**, **dark**, **back**.

- Place a barrier between yourself and the child so that you cannot see each other's pictures. Arrange at least two of your pictures behind the barrier so that the child cannot see what they are. Name the pictures, e.g. '**Fork. Back.**'

- Pause for a few seconds and then say: 'Ready. Steady. Go!' The child listens, then looks at her pictures, finds the ones she heard you name and lays them out on her side of the barrier. When you remove the barrier, you will see if the child's pictures are the same as yours! Reverse the game so that the child names pictures for you to remember and arrange behind the barrier.

- Play *Kim's game* with the small pictures (see the instructions in Section 8, p. 189).

- Play *Pairs* (see the instructions in Section 8, p. 189).

Listen and guess (Listening and speaking activity)

Aim

To say longer words that end with the speech sound **k**: **book, duck, sack, lake, beak, bike, fork, sock, shark, Mark, dark, back, lock, park.**

How?

By giving the child opportunities to hear, and see, you say words that end with **k** and to practise saying the words.

Resources

- Small pictures of words that end with **k** (pp. 119–121).

Instructions

1 Choose a picture, e.g. **bike**. Do not show it to the child. Place it face down in front of her.

2 Tell the child at least three facts about the picture, e.g. 'It has got two wheels. It has got handlebars. You can ride it.'

3 The child guesses what the picture is and turns it over to see if she is right. Reverse the game so that the child chooses a picture and describes it and you guess what it is.

Variations

- To make this activity more challenging for the child, put at least three pictures in front of her, e.g. **bike, book, sock.**

- Choose one of the pictures to describe, e.g. **sock**. Do not tell the child which one you have chosen. Tell her three facts about the picture, e.g. 'You can wear it. It is usually made of wool. You wear it on your foot.'

- To make this activity more challenging, choose at least three pictures. Do not show them to the child. Place them face down in front of her. Tell the child at least three facts about the first picture. The child guesses what it is and turns it over to see if she is correct. Then tell her three facts about the second picture. The child guesses and checks if she is right or not. Follow the same procedure for the third picture. Reverse the game, so that the child chooses at least three pictures and describes them to you.

- Place a barrier between you and the child. Make sure that you and the child each have a set of the small pictures. Choose at least three pictures from your set, e.g. **duck**, **shark**, **lock**. Describe the pictures to the child, leaving a pause between each description so that she can find the picture she thinks you are talking about in her set. When the child has found the picture she thinks you are describing, she puts it face up behind the barrier so that you cannot see it.

- When you have described all three pictures, and the child has put three corresponding pictures behind the barrier, ask her to say what her pictures are, e.g. '**duck**, **shark**, **lock**'. Then remove the barrier to see if she has the same pictures as you. Reverse the game, so that the child chooses and describes her pictures and you listen and try to find the corresponding pictures in your set.

What did I say? (Listening and speaking activity)

Aim

To say longer words that end with the speech sound **k**: **book**, **duck**, **sack**, **lake**, **beak**, **bike**, **fork**, **sock**, **shark**, **Mark**, **dark**, **back**, **lock**, **park**.

How?
By giving the child opportunities to hear, and see, you say longer words that end with **k** and to practise saying the words.

Resources
- At least two sets of the small pictures of words that end with **k** (pp. 119–121).

Instructions

You are the speaker and the child is the listener in this activity.

1   Choose two pictures, e.g. **back** and **dark**. Put them on the table in front of the child and name them for her, e.g. '**Back. Dark.**' Tell the child to listen carefully and then you name one of the pictures placed in front of her, e.g. '**Dark**'. Then say 'What did I say?' The child listens and points to, or holds up, or puts a counter on the word she heard you say.

2   When you think the child is ready to listen and remember more words, choose three pictures, e.g. **book**, **duck** and **fork**. Put them on the table in front of the child and name them for her: '**Book. Duck. Fork.**' Tell the child to listen carefully and then you name two of the pictures placed in front of her, e.g. '**Book. Fork.**' Then say 'What did I say?' The child listens and points to, or holds up, or puts a counter on the words she heard you say. Increase the number of words to make the activity more challenging when you think the child is ready. For example, choose four pictures, name them, then name three of the four and ask the child to point to the three which you said.

Variations

* To make the activity more challenging, present at least three pictures to the child. Write down the words in the order you are going to say them, not in the order they are in front of the child. For example, if the pictures in front of the child are **park**, **Mark**, **shark**, you might write down **shark**, **park**, **Mark**. Read out the words that you have written down: '**Shark. Park. Mark.**' The child listens and arranges the pictures correspondingly, i.e. to match what you said (**shark**, **park**, **Mark**). To do this activity, the child needs to be able to write, but not spell!

* Give the same pictures to yourself and to the child. You will need at least three, e.g. **bike**, **lock**, **sack**. Place a barrier between yourself and the child so that you cannot see each other's pictures. Arrange your pictures without the child seeing. Name the pictures in the order you have arranged them, e.g. '**Sock. Bike. Lock.** ' The child listens and arranges her pictures to match what you have said. Remove the barrier and see if the child's pictures are in the same order as yours! Reverse the game so that the child is the speaker and you are the listener.

What's the word? (Listening activity)

Aim

To say longer words that end with the speech sound **k**: **book, duck, sack, lake, beak, bike, fork, sock, shark, Mark, dark, back, lock, park**.

How?

By giving the child opportunities to hear, and see, you say words that end with **k** and to practise saying the words.

Resources

- At least two sets of the small pictures of words that end with **k** (pp. 119–121).

Instructions

This activity is for children aged four and a half upwards.

1 Put at least four small pictures in front of the child. Name them with the child, e.g. '**Beak. Duck. Lake. Shark**', so that she can hear the words before you start the activity.

2 Tell the child to listen carefully and point to the picture you are naming. Break the words into two parts, e.g. **bea – k, du – ck, la – ke, shar – k**. Leave a short pause between the two parts of the words to help the child carry out this task. The child has to put the speech sounds together in her head to make the word, e.g. **beak**, and then point to the picture of a beak.

3 When the child is familiar with this activity, ask her to put the sounds together in her head, e.g. **du – ck**, point to the picture and say the word out loud, e.g. '**duck**'.

Variations

- Give one set of the small pictures to yourself and one to the child. Choose at least three. Do not show the child the pictures you have chosen. Place a barrier between yourself and the child so that you cannot see each other's pictures.

- Arrange your pictures without the child seeing them on your side of the barrier, e.g. **park, lock, fork**. Tell the child to listen carefully, find the pictures you say and put them on her side of the barrier. Sound the words out, leaving a pause before the **k** at the end of each word, e.g. '**Par – k. Lo – ck. For – k.**' The child has to put the speech sounds together in her head, find the picture and put it behind her barrier. When you have finished, ask the child to say what the pictures are, e.g. '**Park. Lock. Fork.**' Remove the barrier to see if they are the same as your pictures.

- Challenge older children by breaking words into three parts, e.g. **p – ar – k, l – o – ck, f – or – k**.

Tips

*How can I help the child to say **k** at the end of words?*

You will need two coins or Lego bricks and small pictures of the words that you are working on with the child, e.g. **back**, **bike**, **duck**. Choose one of the pictures, e.g. **back**. Put the two coins or bricks in front of the child, leaving a gap between the two objects. Touch the first coin or brick and say the first part of the word, e.g. **ba**. Then touch the second coin or brick and say the final speech sound, e.g. **k** (**ba – k**). Take it in turns to touch the coins or bricks and say **ba** and **k** as you touch each one. Gradually move the two objects closer together so that the pause you leave between saying **ba** and saying **k** is smaller and smaller, until the coins or bricks are touching and there is no gap between **ba** and **k**, i.e. you are saying **back**.

My progress

Date	I can ...	☺/☹	I need to work on ...
	Listen carefully and hear words that end with **k**, e.g. **back**, **bike**, **duck**, without any help.		
	Listen carefully and hear words that end with **k**, e.g. **back**, **bike**, **duck**, with help.		
	Say **k** at the end of words, e.g. **back**, **bike**, **duck**, without any help.		
	Say **k** at the end of words, e.g. **back**, **bike**, **duck**, with some help.		

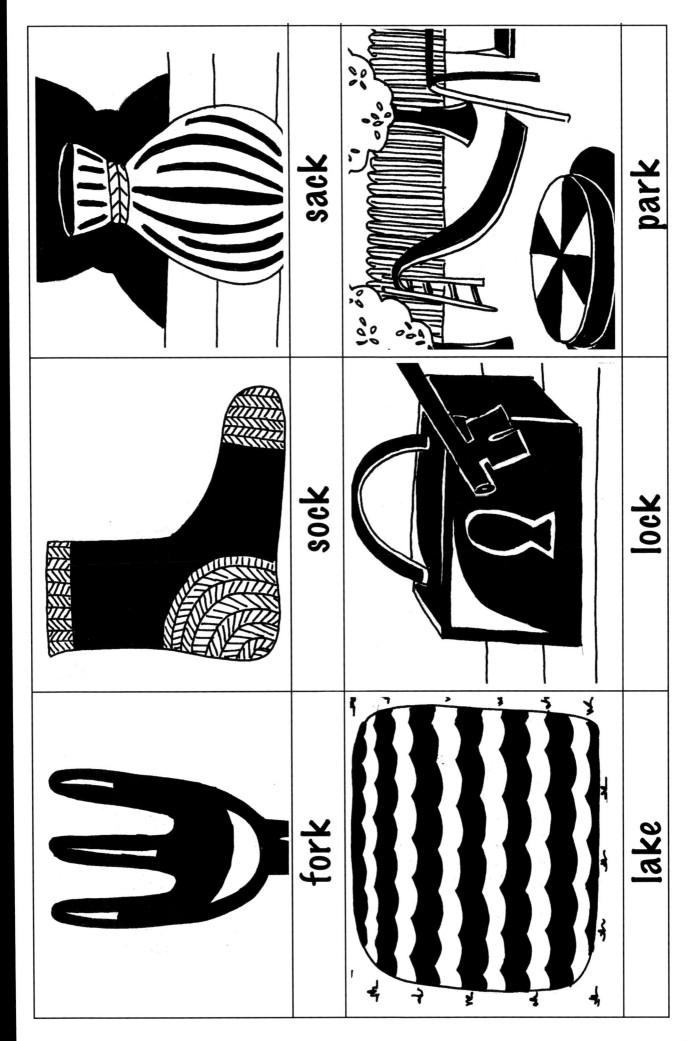

sack

park

sock

lock

fork

lake

119

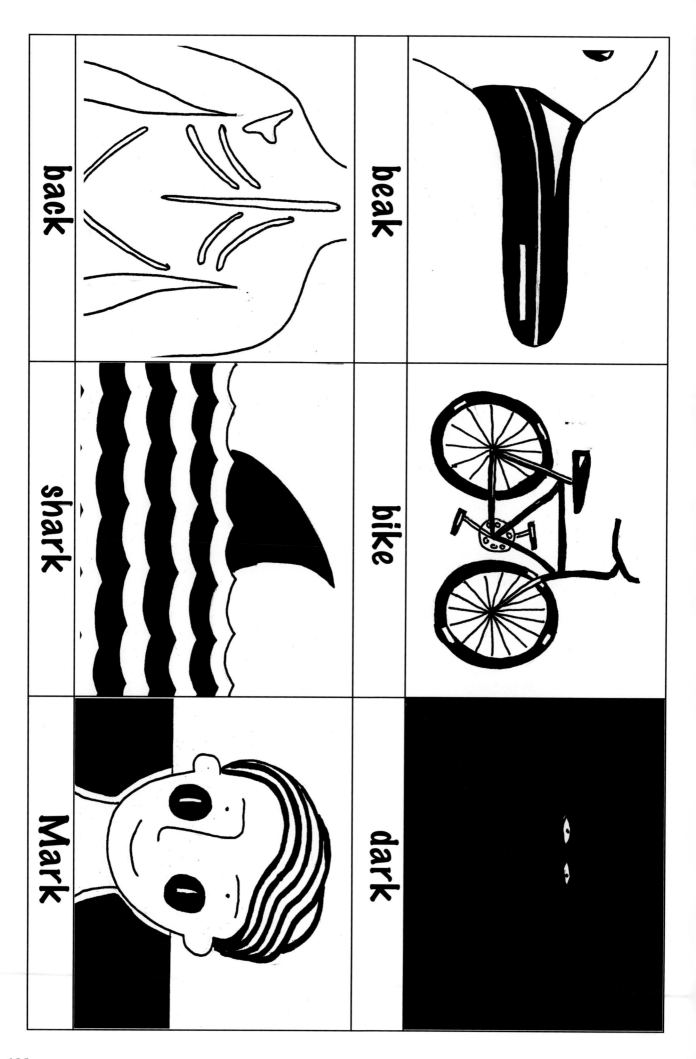

beak

back

bike

shark

dark

Mark

book

duck

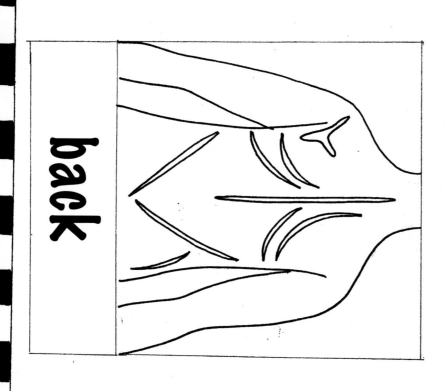

back

dark

Look!

Look!

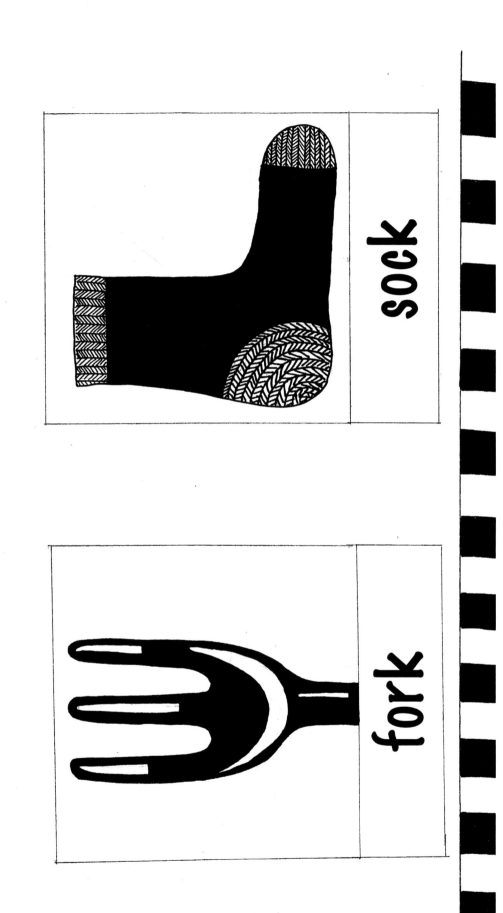

fork

sock

shark

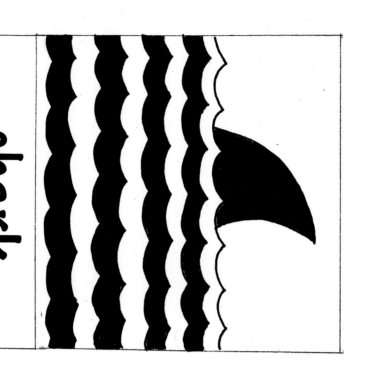

Mark

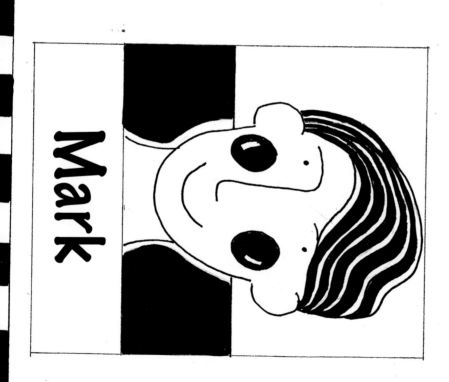

Look!

Look!

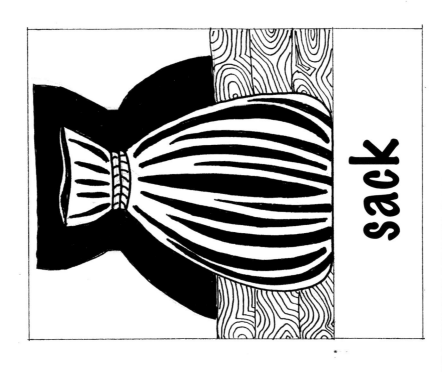

sack

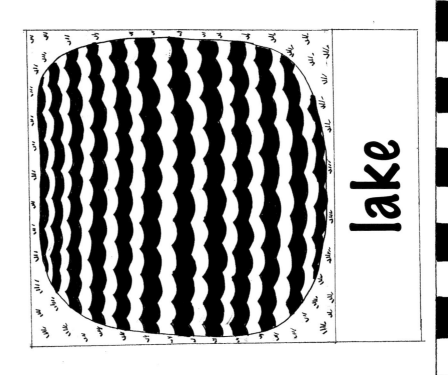

lake

Look!

bike

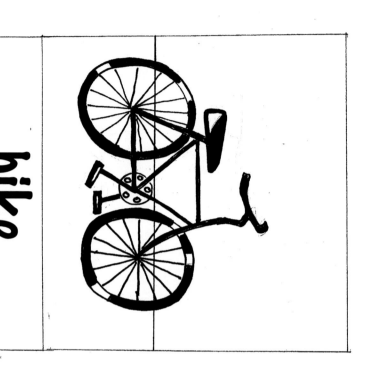

beak

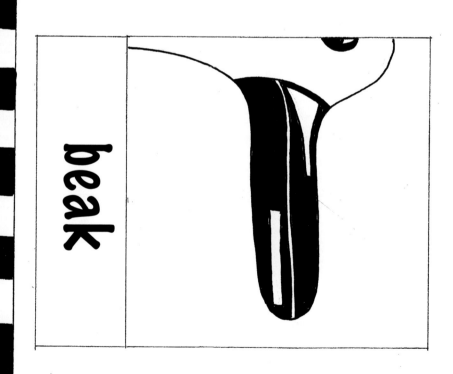

Look!

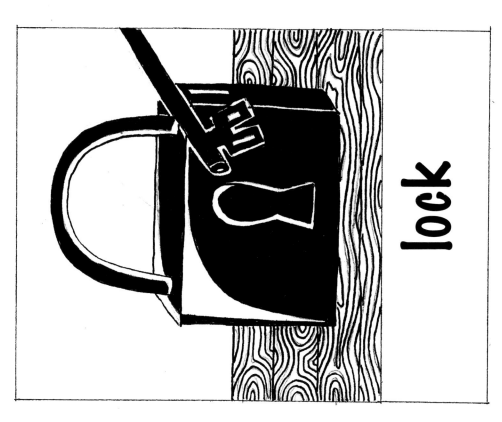

lock

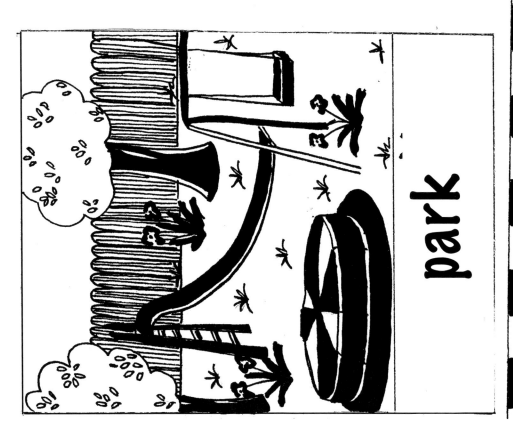

park

duck

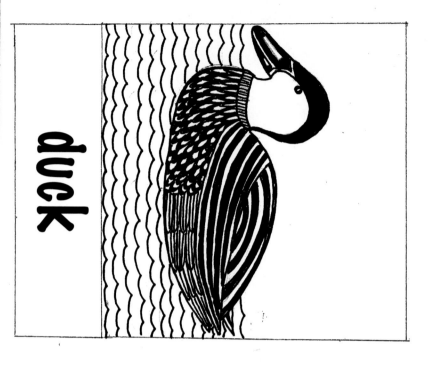

book

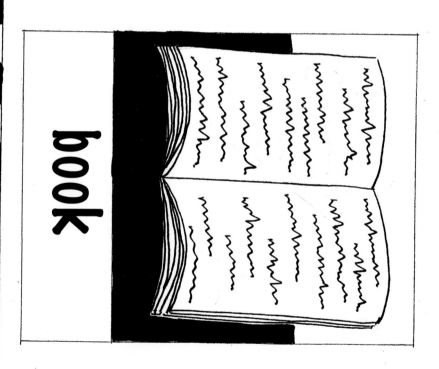

Look!

What's the next step?

- I can listen carefully and hear words that end with **k**, e.g. **back**, **bike**, **duck**, without any help. **Continue to play listening games from the list of games in Section 8. Start working on Section 6.**

- I can listen carefully and hear words that end with **k**, e.g. **back**, **bike**, **duck**, with help. **Keep playing listening games from Section 5. Play listening games from earlier sections to revise listening to k in words and listening games from the list of games in Section 8, e.g. Listen and do. When the child can hear words that end with k 70 per cent of the time in listening games, start working on listening games in Section 6.**

- I can say **k** at the end of words, e.g. **back**, **bike**, **duck**, without any help. **Start working on speaking activities in Section 6. Play speaking games from the list of games in Section 8, e.g. Pairs, Kim's game.**

- I can say **k** at the end of words, e.g. **back**, **bike**, **duck**, with some help. **Continue doing speaking activities from Section 5. Play speaking games from the list of games in Section 8. When the child can say words that end with k 70 per cent of the time in speaking games, start working on listening games in Section 6.**

Jingles with words that end with k

See the advice at the end of Section 3 on how to use the jingles in sessions (pp. 64–65).

Jingle 1   (pictures on p. 132)

Listen

Red sock

Yellow sock

Pink sock

Purple sock

Stripey sock

Spotty sock

Which sock shall I wear?

Say the word

Red _____ (sock)

Yellow _____ (sock)

Pink _____ (sock)

Purple _____ (sock)

Stripey _____ (sock)

Spotty _____ (sock)

Which _____ (sock) shall I wear?

Jingle 2   (pictures on p. 133)

Listen

On Monday, I saw a duck riding a bike!

On Tuesday, I saw a duck reading a book!

On Wednesday, I saw a duck eating with a fork!

On Thursday, I saw a duck washing a sock!

On Friday, I saw a duck swimming with a shark!

I never saw the duck again!

Say the word

On Monday, I saw a duck riding a _____ (bike)!

On Tuesday, I saw a duck reading a _____ (book)!

On Wednesday, I saw a duck eating with a _____ (fork)!

On Thursday, I saw a duck washing a _____ (sock)!

On Friday, I saw a duck swimming with a _____ (shark)!

I never saw the duck again!

Jingle 3   (pictures on p. 135)

Listen

Knock, knock

Who's there?

Open the door and see!

Quack, quack!

It's a duck

Ssssss!

It's a snake

Say the word

Knock, _____ (knock)

Who's there?

Open the door and see!

Quack, _____ (quack)!

It's a _____ (duck)

Ssssss!

It's a _____ (snake)

Jingle 4   (pictures on p. 134)

Listen

I went for a walk in the park

I went for a walk in the dark

I went for a ride on my bike

I went for a ride with my friend Mike

I had a bath with a shark

Who can sing like a lark

Say the word

I went for a walk in the _____ (park)

I went for a walk in the _____ (dark)

I went for a ride on my _____ (bike)

I went for a ride with my friend _____ (Mike)

I had a bath with a _____ (shark)

Who can sing like a _____ (lark)

Which sock shall I wear?

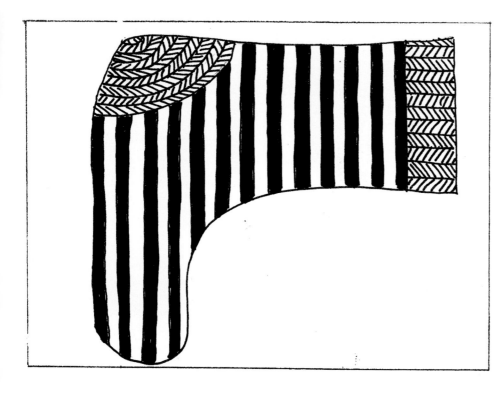

A stripey sock

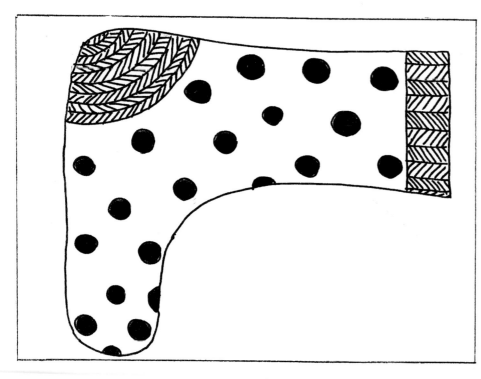

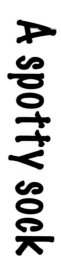

A spotty sock

A duck swimming with a shark

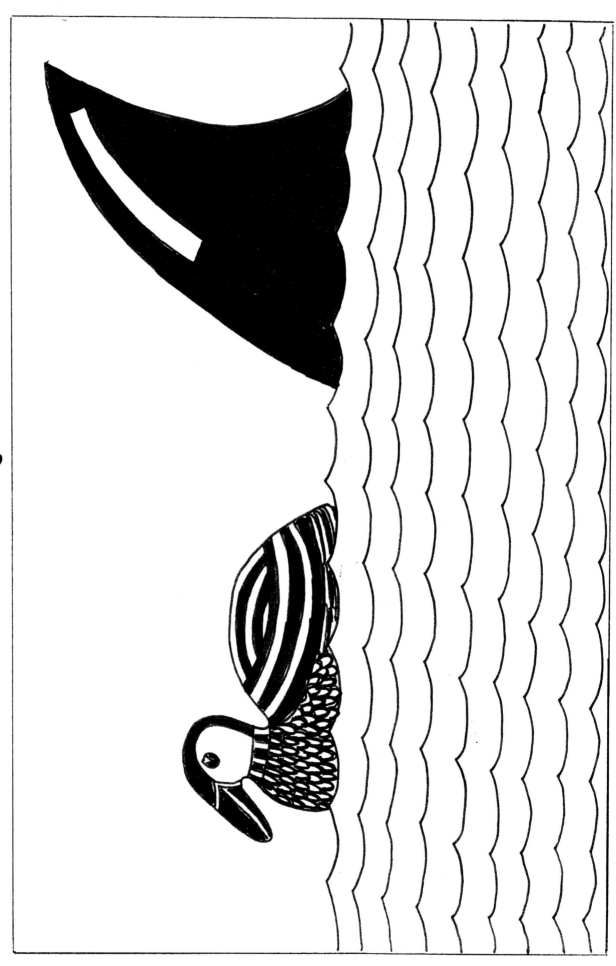

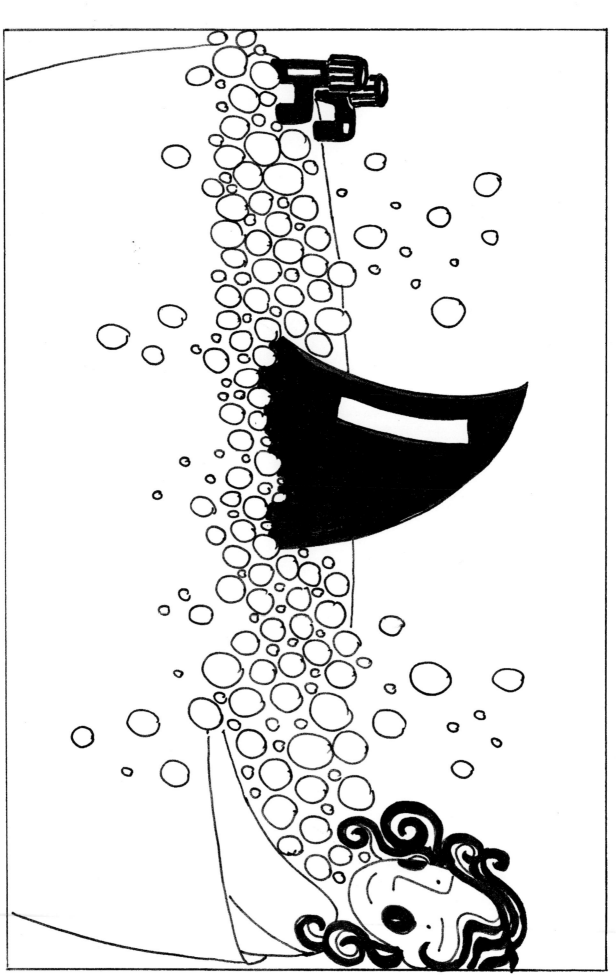

A bath with a shark

Knock, knock!

sssss!

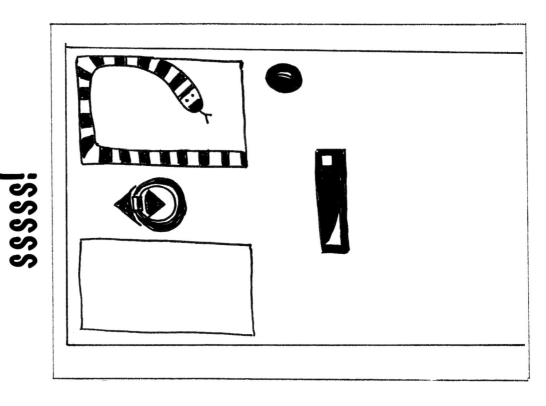

Quack, quack!

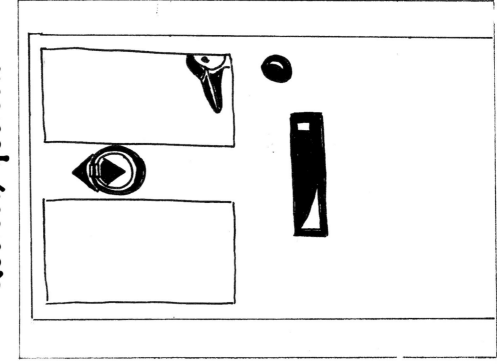

SAYING K AT THE BEGINNING OF WORDS WITH MORE THAN ONE SYLLABLE

Section 6: **Saying k at the beginning of words with more than one syllable**

What's the picture? (Speaking activity)

Aim

To say longer words that begin with the speech sound **k** and have more than one syllable: **cooker, cowboy, coffee, kipper, kettle, cuckoo, camel, candle, carrot, comic, kitten, kitchen, kangaroo, cupboard, carpet, cushion, cauliflower, coconut, cucumber, caterpillar**.

How?

By giving the child opportunities to hear, and see, you say longer words that begin with **k** and to practise saying the words.

Resources

- Large pictures of words that begin with **k** and have more than one syllable (pp. 146–155).

- Small pictures of words that begin with **k** and have more than one syllable (pp. 157–159).

- Page of two doors with question marks on each one and the instruction *What's the picture?* (p. 64). You will need to photocopy this page and cut along three sides of the doors so that you can open them to reveal a picture.

Instructions

1 Put the page with the doors on top of large pictures of words that begin with **k**, e.g. **coffee** and **kangaroo**.

2 Read the instruction at the top of the page to the child: *What's the picture? Open the door and see.* Before you open the door to see what the picture is, say: 'My turn!' so that the child knows you are going first. Open the first door to reveal the picture and name it, e.g. 'Look! **Coffee**!' so that the child has an opportunity to hear you say **k** at the beginning of a short word.

3 When you have finished your go, say to the child: 'Your turn!' so that he knows that it is his go to open the door and name the picture behind it.

4 Put the picture of the doors over different large pictures, e.g. **kitten** and **cucumber**, and take it in turns to open a door and name the picture behind it. Follow this procedure to name all the large pictures on the pages for this activity.

Variation

- Tell the child to close his eyes and put a small picture of a word beginning with **k** behind each door. Then ask the child to open his eyes and open the doors. Try asking him to guess what picture is behind the door before he opens it.

Look and guess (Speaking activity)

Aim

To say longer words that begin with the speech sound **k** and have more than one syllable: **cooker, cowboy, coffee, kipper, kettle, cuckoo, camel, candle, carrot, comic, kitten, kitchen, kangaroo, cupboard, carpet, cushion, cauliflower, coconut, cucumber, caterpillar**.

How

By giving the child opportunities to hear, and see, you say longer words that begin with **k** and to practise saying the words.

Resources

- Two pictures of magnifying glasses (p. 161). Each magnifying glass has a hole in the lens. Cut out each magnifying glass and cut out the hole on each.

- Large pictures of longer words that begin with **k** and have more than one syllable (pp. 146–155).

Instructions

1 Make sure the child cannot see the pictures, e.g. **cooker** and **cowboy**. Cover one of the pictures with the magnifying glass which has the smaller hole so that a bit of the picture can be seen through the hole.

2 Let the child have two or three guesses at what the picture is. If he cannot guess, change magnifying glasses so that the hole in the lens is bigger and more of the picture can be seen through it. Then ask the child what he thinks the picture is.

Tips

*Help! The child says **gamel** instead of **camel**! What can I do?*

- Break the word into two halves, e.g. **ca** and **mel**. Leave a pause between the two halves, e.g. **ca** (pause) **mel**. Gradually make the pause that you leave between the two halves of the word smaller until there is no pause and you are saying the word: '**camel**'. Try some of the ideas described in the tips to help the child say longer words that start with **k** (Section 4, p. 86) , e.g. **can**. For example: put two paper hands on the wall. Touch a hand and say **ca**. Touch the other hand and say **mel**. Gradually bring the hands closer together, making the pause between **ca** and **mel** smaller.

When the child is ready, put the hands next to each other and say the word without a pause: '**camel**'.

Help! I have tried these tips and the child still finds it hard to say longer words! He gets all the sounds muddled up! What can I do?

- It takes some children longer than others to say words. Children need to hear words many times in order to say them correctly. They need lots of opportunities to practise saying the words you are working on, e.g. **cupboard**, in activities and games. Regular repetition is important. Carry out work at the child's pace.

Finish my word (Speaking activity)

Aim
To say longer words that begin with the speech sound **k** and have more than one syllable: **cooker, cowboy, coffee, kipper, kettle, cuckoo, camel, candle, carrot, comic, kitten, kitchen, kangaroo, cupboard, carpet, cushion, cauliflower, coconut, cucumber, caterpillar**.

How?
By giving the child opportunities to hear, and see, you say longer words that begin with **k** and to practise saying the words.

Resources
- Two sets of the small pictures of longer words that begin with **k** and have more than one syllable (pp. 157–159).

Instructions
This activity is for children aged four and a half upwards.

1 Put at least three pictures in a line in front of the child, e.g. **cooker, cuckoo, coffee**. Tell the child that you have a really bad memory and can't remember the ends of words. Ask the child if he can help you name the pictures.

2 Say the first syllable of each word, e.g. '**Coo___**. Oh, what is it? **Coo___**. I know it, I just can't quite remember it! **Coo___**. It's no good I can't remember it! Can you help me?' See if the child can complete the word (**cooker**). If he says '**ker**', say the word aloud,

e.g. '**Cooker**! Of course! Thanks' and then ask him to say it for you, e.g. 'Oh, no! I've forgotten it again! Can you help me again, please? What is it?'

Variations

- Put at least three pictures in front of the child. Ask him to listen carefully and point to the picture that you say, or put a counter on it, or hold it up. Break the word into syllables, leaving a pause between the syllables, e.g. '**Coo – ker**'.

- Choose at least five pictures. Make sure the child has the same pictures that you have. Place a barrier between you and the child so that you cannot see each other's pictures. Say at least two words for the child, breaking the words into syllables, e.g. **coo – ker, co – ffee**.' The child listens, and arranges his pictures on his side of the barrier in the order he hears them. Ask the child what pictures he has so that he has to name them for you. Then remove the barrier to see if they match your pictures.

What did I say? (Listening and speaking activity)

Aim

To say longer words that begin with the speech sound **k** and have more than one syllable: **cooker, cowboy, coffee, kipper, kettle, cuckoo, camel, candle, carrot, comic, kitten, kitchen, kangaroo, cupboard, carpet, cushion, cauliflower, coconut, cucumber, caterpillar**.

How?

By giving the child opportunities to hear, and see, you say longer words that begin with **k** and to practise saying the words.

Resources

- At least two sets of the small pictures of longer words that begin with **k** and have more than one syllable (pp. 157–159).

Instructions

You are the speaker and the child is the listener in these activities.

1 Choose two pictures, e.g. **carrot** and **kitten**. Put them on the table in front of the child and name them for him: '**Carrot. Kitten**'. Tell the child to listen carefully and then you name one of the pictures placed in front of him, e.g. '**Carrot**'. Then say 'What did I say?' The child listens and points to, or holds up, or puts a counter on the picture of the word he heard you say.

2 When you think the child is ready to listen and remember more words, choose three pictures, e.g. **comic**, **cuckoo** and **coconut**. Put them on the table in front of the child and name them for him: '**Comic. Cuckoo. Coconut.**' Tell the child to listen carefully and then name two of the pictures placed in front of him, e.g. '**Coconut. Comic.**' Then say 'What did I say?' The child listens and points to, or holds up, or puts a counter on the words he heard you say. Increase the number of words to make the activity more challenging when you think the child is ready. For example, choose four pictures, name them, then name three of the four and ask the child to point to the three that you said.

Variations

- To make the activity more challenging, present at least three pictures to the child. Write down the words in the order you are going to say them, not in the order they are in front of the child. For example, if the pictures in front of the child are **kipper**, **candle**, **kitten**, you might write down **candle**, **kitten**, **kipper**. Read out the words that you have written down: '**Candle. Kitten. Kipper.**' The child listens and arranges the pictures correspondingly, i.e. to match what you said (**candle**, **kitten**, **kipper**). To do this activity, the child needs to be able to write, but not spell!

- Give the same pictures to yourself and to the child. You will need at least three, e.g. **comic**, **kitchen**, **camel**. Place a barrier between yourself and the child so that you cannot see each other's pictures. Arrange your pictures without the child seeing. Name the pictures in the order you have arranged them, e.g. '**Camel. Comic. Kitchen.**' The child listens and arranges his pictures to match what you have said. Remove the barrier and see if the child's pictures are in the same order as yours! Reverse the game so that the child is the speaker and you are the listener.

Roll and say (Speaking activity)

Aim

To say longer words that begin with the speech sound **k** and have more than one syllable: **cooker**, **cowboy**, **coffee**, **kipper**, **kettle**, **cuckoo**, **camel**, **candle**, **carrot**, **comic**, **kitten**, **kitchen**, **kangaroo**, **cupboard**, **carpet**, **cushion**, **cauliflower**, **coconut**, **cucumber**, **caterpillar**.

How?

By giving the child opportunities to hear, and see, you say longer words that begin with **k** and to practise saying the words.

Resources

- A set of the small pictures (pp. 157–159) that have shapes on the back (photocopy the sheet of shapes (p. 28) onto the back of the pictures).

- A dice

- The template for a dice with a different shape on each face (p. 30).

Instructions

1. Spread out the pictures in front of the child, face down, so that you cannot see the pictures but you can see the shapes on the back.

2. Roll the dice with shapes on it. The shapes on the dice match the shapes on the back of the pictures. Turn over the picture that has the same shape as the dice, e.g. circle, so that you can see what the picture is, e.g. **candle**.

3. Roll the dice with numbers on it. You have to say the word on your picture, e.g. **candle**, the number of times that you throw on the dice, e.g. five: '**candle, candle, candle, candle, candle**.' Make sure you have the first turn so that you can demonstrate the activity to the child.

Variations

- Make the game competitive: the winner is the first person to say the names of all of the six pictures in the activity, i.e. to throw all of the shapes on the dice.

- Roll the dice with shapes on it and turn over the picture that has the same shape on it, e.g. a heart. Take it in turns to see how many times you can say the word in a minute. Use a one-minute salt timer.

My progress

Date	I can ...	☺/☹	I need to work on ...
	Listen carefully and hear long words that begin with **k**, e.g. **cooker**, **camel**, **carpet**, without any help.		
	Listen carefully and hear long words that begin with **k**, e.g. **cooker**, **camel**, **carpet**, with help.		
	Say **k** at the beginning of long words, e.g. **cooker**, **camel**, **carpet**, without any help.		
	Say **k** at the beginning of long words, e.g. **cooker**, **camel**, **carpet**, with some help.		

Look!

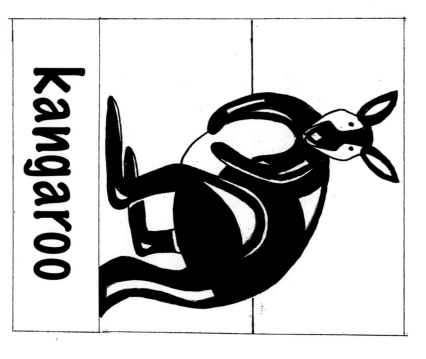

kangaroo

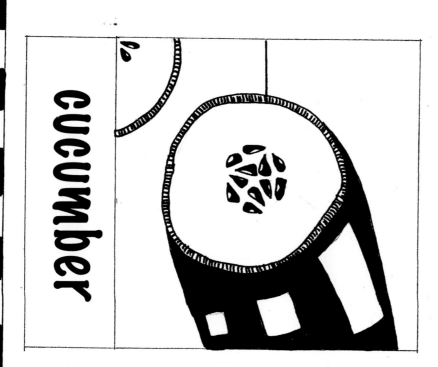

cucumber

Look!

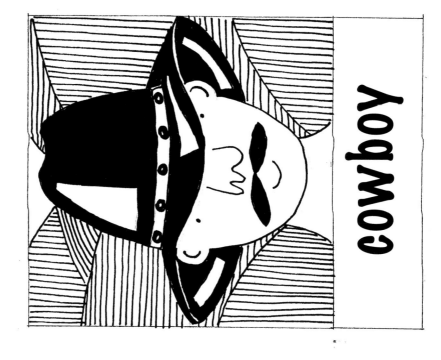

cowboy

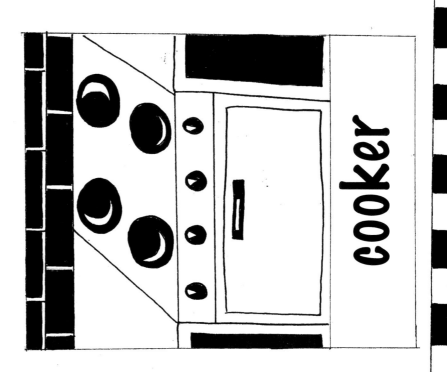

cooker

Look!

kettle

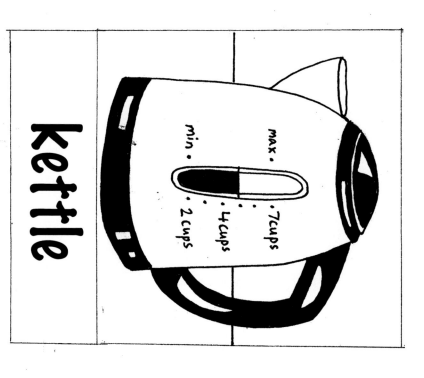

max.
min.
7cups
4cups
2cups

comic

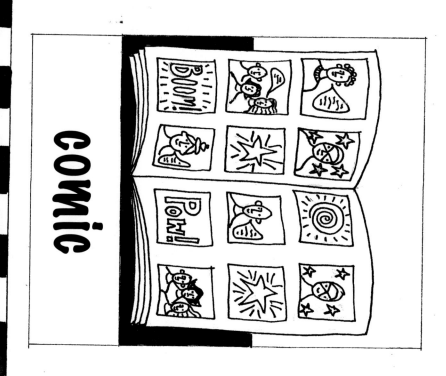

Look!

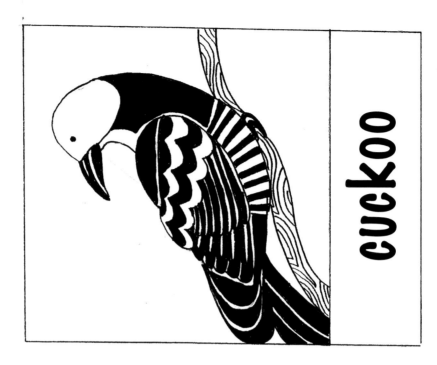

cuckoo

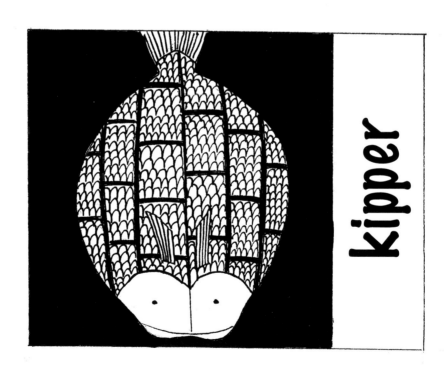

kipper

149

Look!

cushion

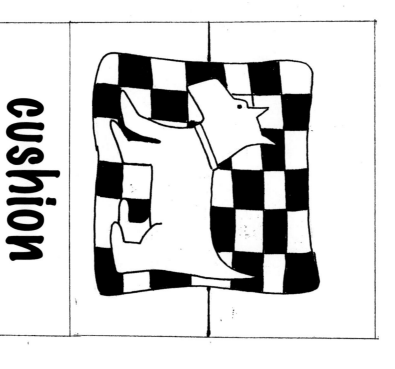

carrot

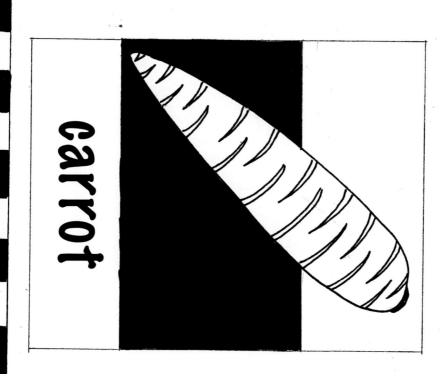

Look!

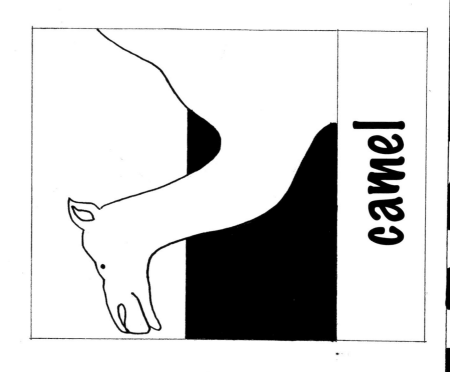

camel

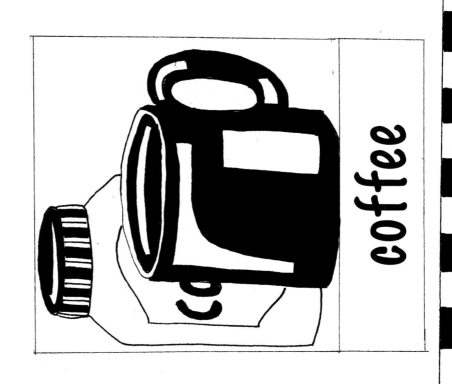

coffee

151

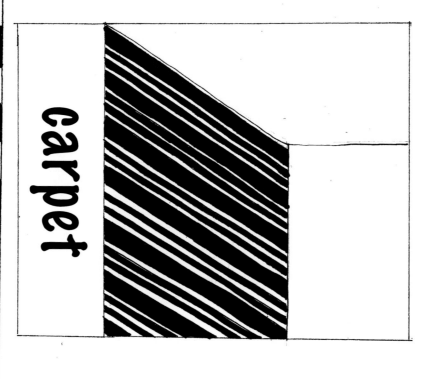

carpet

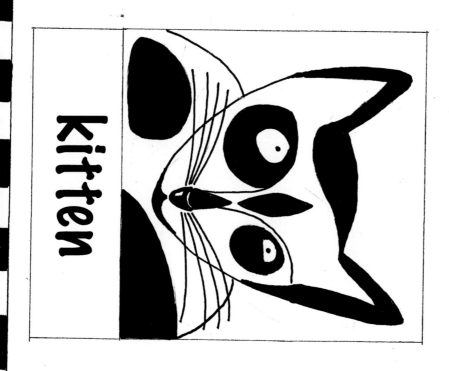

kitten

Look!

Look!

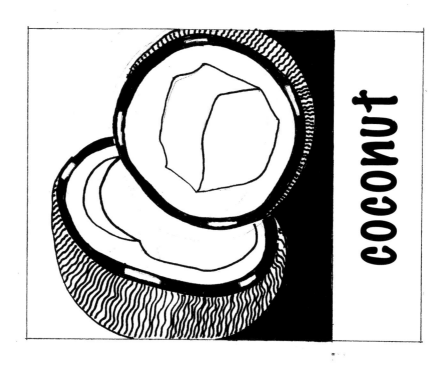

coconut

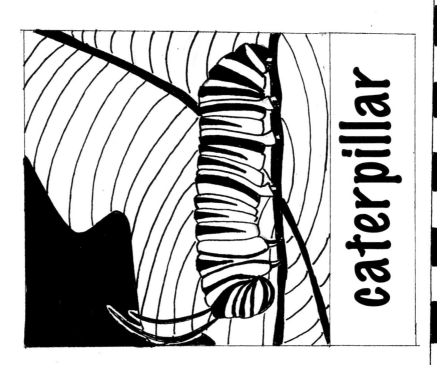

caterpillar

153

Look!

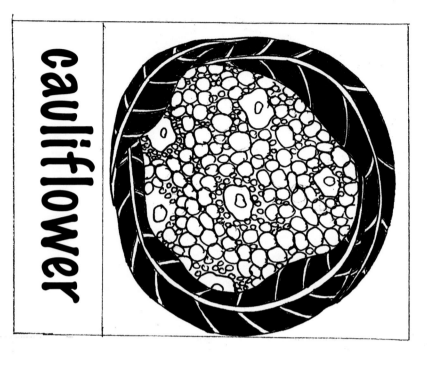

cauliflower

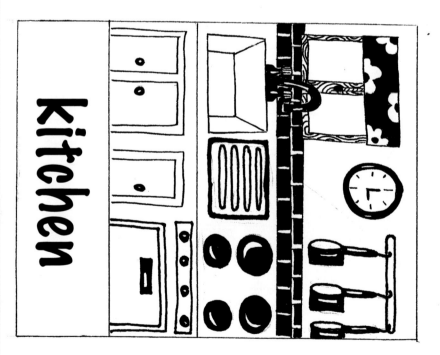

kitchen

Look!

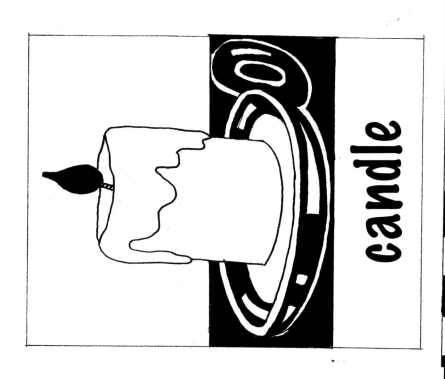

candle

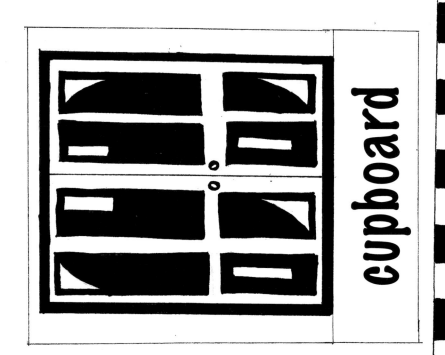

cupboard

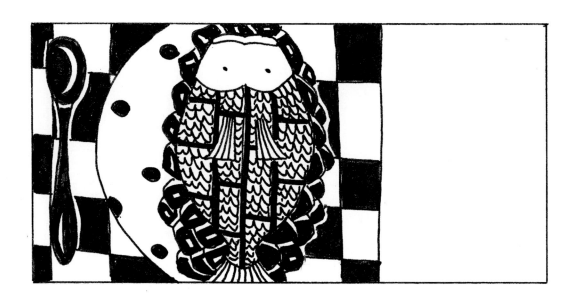

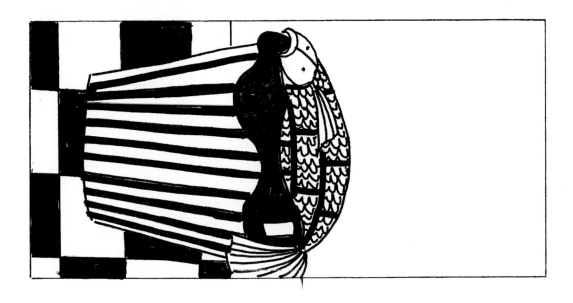

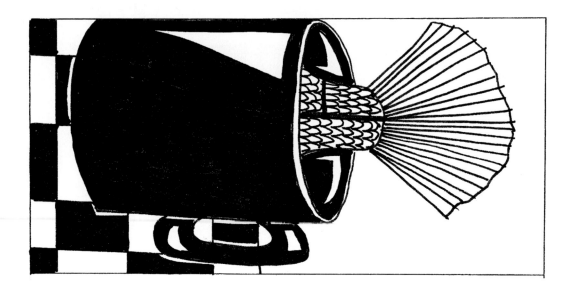

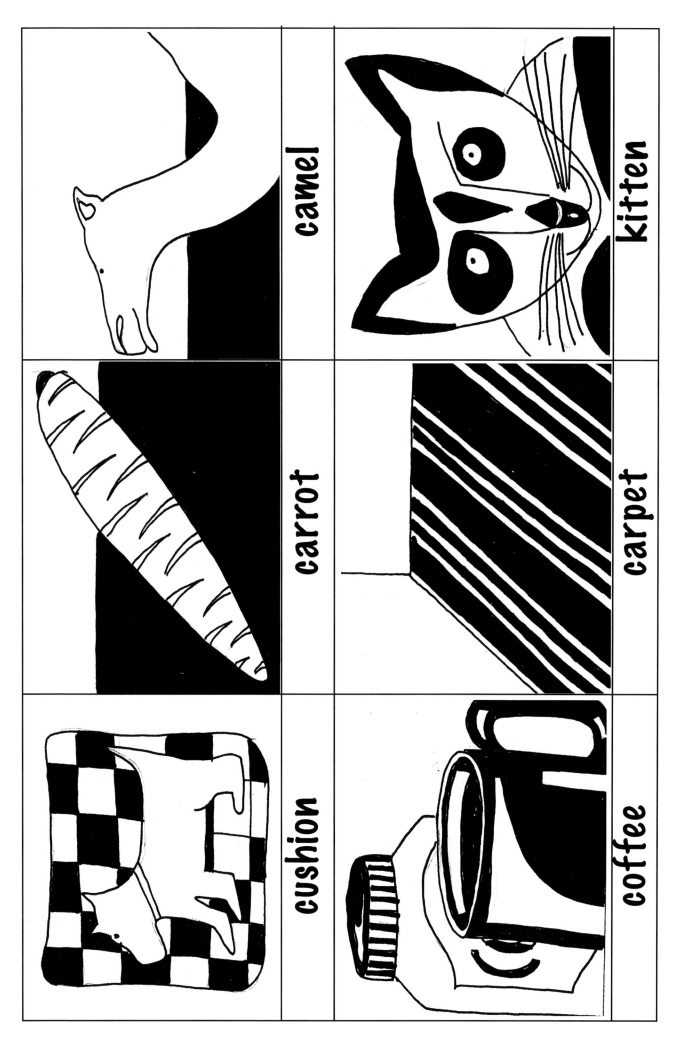

camel

kitten

carrot

carpet

cushion

coffee

157

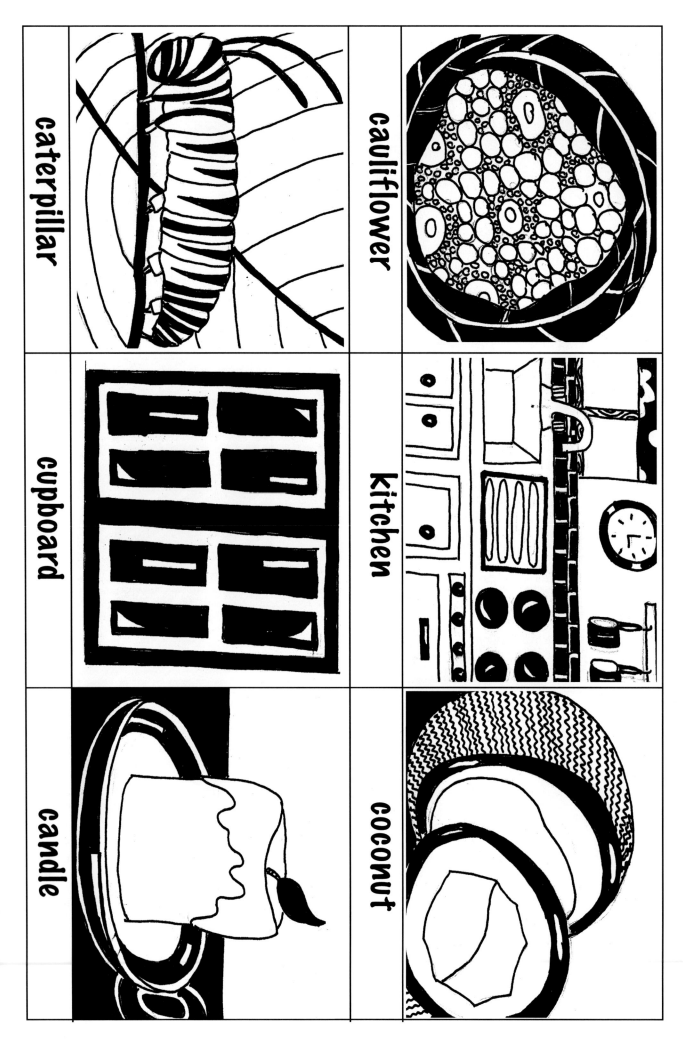

caterpillar

cauliflower

cupboard

kitchen

candle

coconut

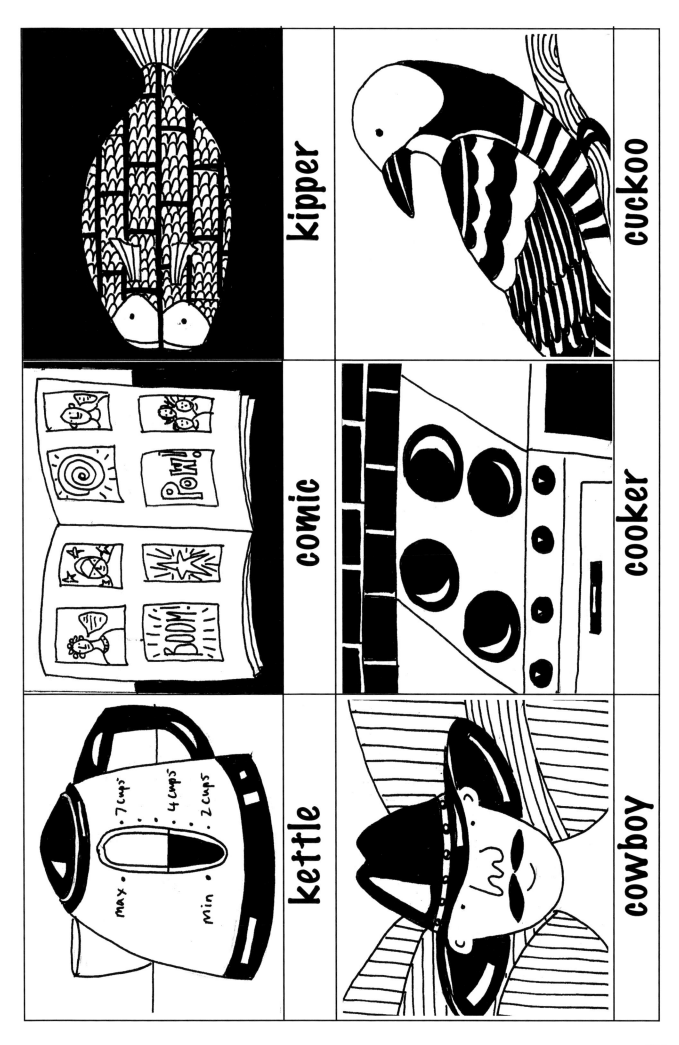

kipper

cuckoo

comic

cooker

kettle

cowboy

159

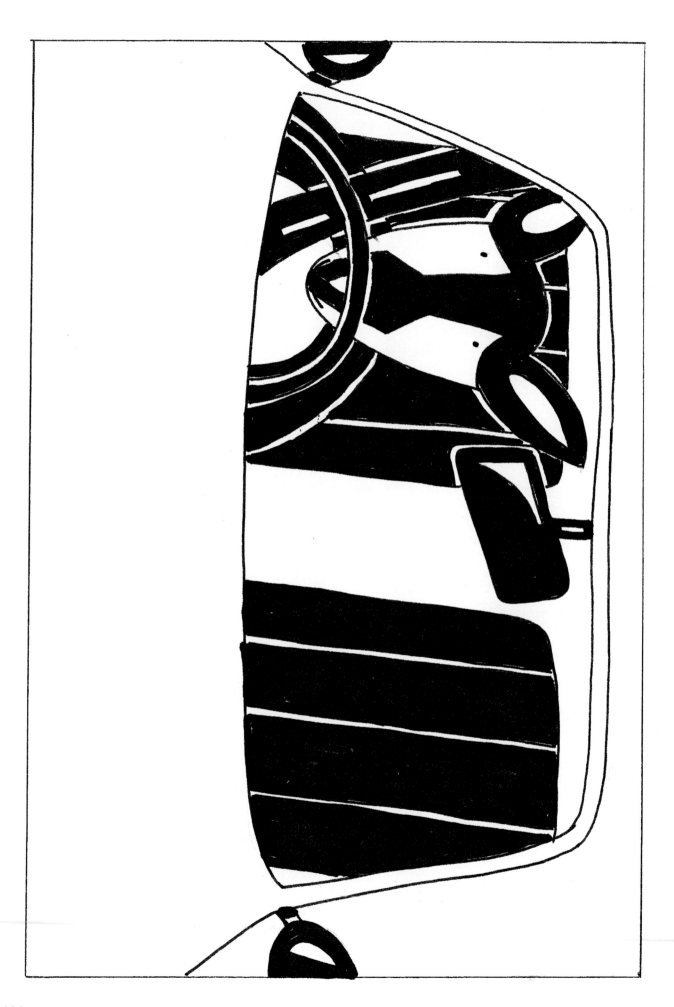

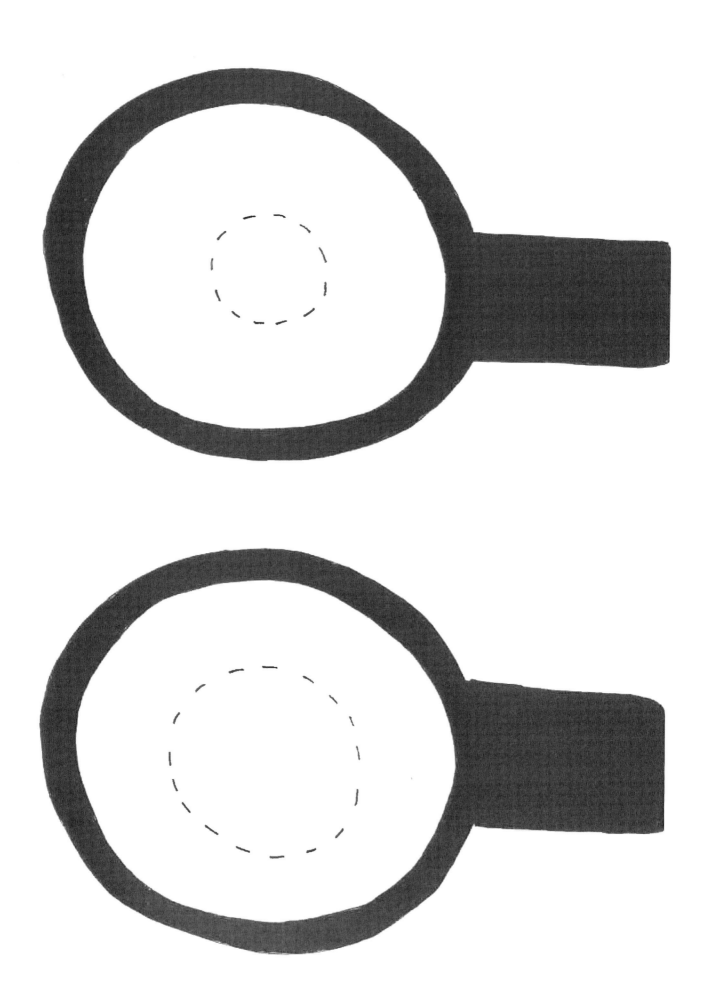

161

What's the next step?

- I can listen carefully and hear long words that begin with **k**, e.g. **cooker**, **camel**, **carpet**, without any help. **Start working on Section 7. Continue playing listening games from the list of games in Section 8.**

- I can listen carefully and hear long words that begin with **k**, e.g. **cooker**, **camel**, **carpet**, with help. **Continue doing listening activities from Section 6. Do listening activities from earlier sections to review work you have done with the child. Play listening games from the list of games in Section 8. When the child can hear long words that begin with k at least 70 per cent of the time in listening activities, start working on Section 7.**

- I can say **k** at the beginning of long words, e.g. **cooker**, **camel**, **carpet**, without any help. **Start working on Section 7. Continue playing speaking games from the list of games in Section 8.**

- I can say **k** at the beginning of long words, e.g. **cooker**, **camel**, **carpet**, with some help. **Continue doing speaking activities from Section 6. Do speaking activities from earlier sections to review work you have done with the child. Play speaking games from the list of games in Section 8. When the child can say long words that begin with k at least 70 per cent of the time in activities, start working on Section 7.**

Jingles with words that begin with k

See the advice at the end of Section 3 on how to use the jingles in sessions (pp. 64–65).

Jingle 1 (pictures on p. 156)

Listen

Would you like a kipper on your cornflakes?

No, thank you

Would you like a kipper on your cupcake?

No, thank you

Would you like a kipper in your coffee?

No, thank you. I don't like kippers

Say the word

Would you like a _____ (kipper) on your cornflakes?

No, thank you

Would you like a kipper on your _____ (cupcake)?

No, thank you

Would you like a kipper in your _____ (coffee)?

No, thank you. I don't like kippers

Jingle 2 (pictures on pp. 150, 151, 153, 154, 165)

Listen

Let's make a cake!

What shall we put in it?

Cucumber and carrot!

Cauliflower and coffee!

Kangaroo and coconut!

Would you like a piece?

No, thank you!

Say the word

Let's make a _____ (cake)!

What shall we put in it?

Cucumber and _____ (carrot)!

Cauliflower and _____ (coffee)!

Kangaroo and _____ (coconut)!

Would you like a piece?

No, thank you!

Jingle 3   (picture on p. 160, 166, 167)

Listen

There's a camel in the kitchen

There's a cowboy in the cupboard

There's a kitten in the kettle

There's a caterpillar on the cushion

There's a kangaroo in the car

It's like living in a zoo!

Say the word

There's a _____ (camel) in the kitchen

There's a _____ (cowboy) in the cupboard

There's a _____ (kitten) in the kettle

There's a _____ (caterpillar) on the cushion

There's a _____ (kangaroo) in the car

It's like living in a zoo!

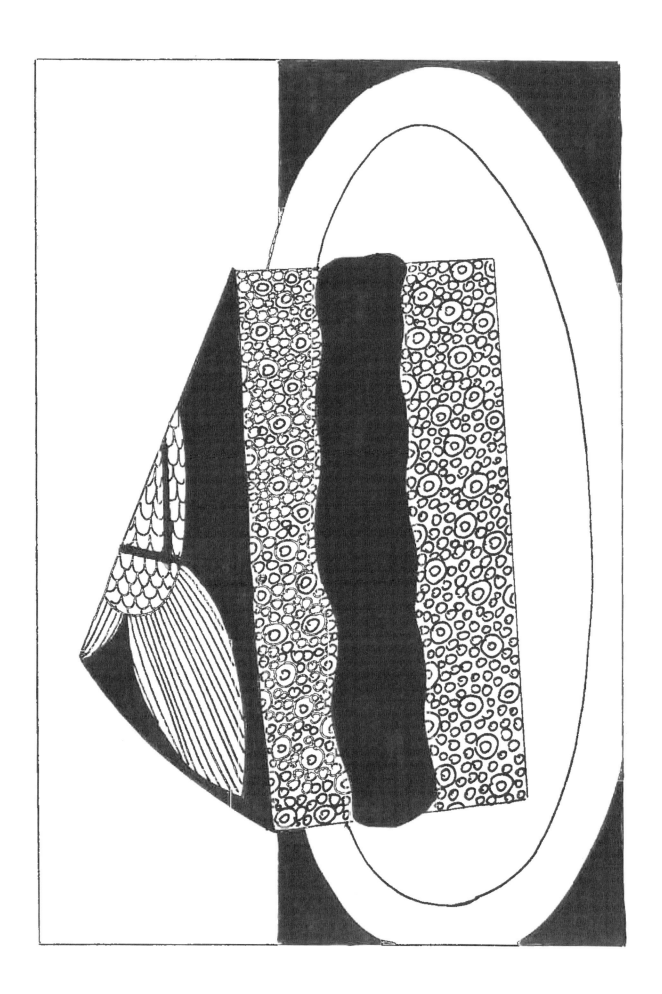

165

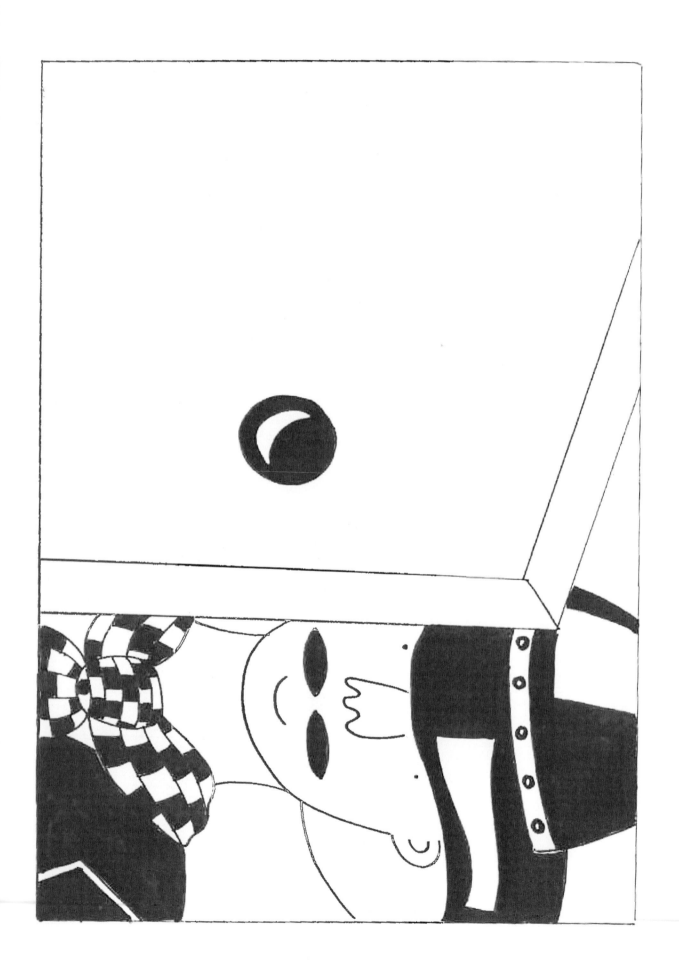

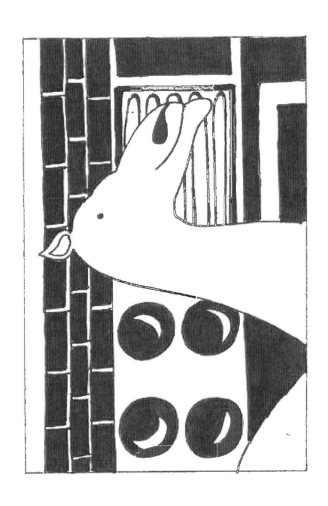

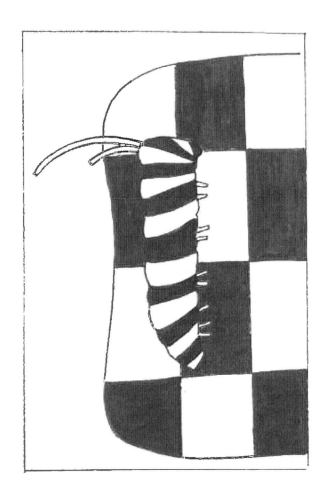

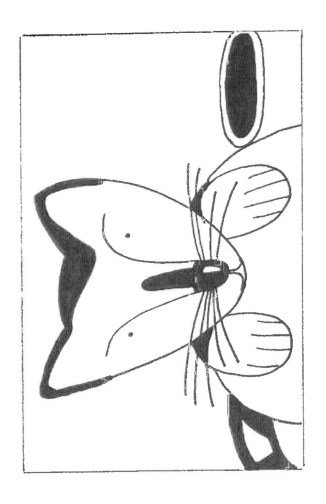

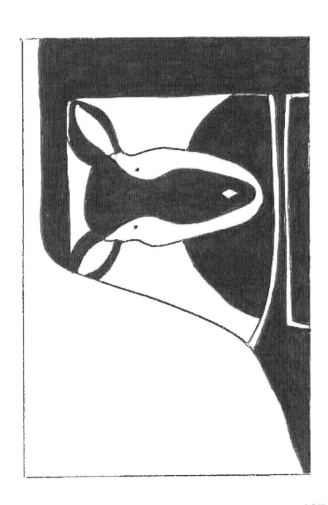

SECTION 7

SAYING K IN PHRASES AND SENTENCES

Section 7: Saying k in phrases and sentences

General advice

Choose which words you want to use in games. For example, you could start playing games using short words that begin with **k** (**car, key, Kai, Kay, cow, core**), then with longer words that begin with **k** (**comb, corn, cup, cap, cat, kite, cake, cook, card, coat, Ken, Kate, coal, cork, can, curl, kiss, case**), then with longer words that end with **k** (**book, duck, sack, lake, beak, bike, fork, sock, shark, Mark, dark, back, lock, park**), and then with words with more than one syllable (**cooker, cowboy, coffee, kipper, kettle, cuckoo, camel, candle, carrot, comic, kitten, kitchen, kangaroo, cupboard, carpet, cushion, cauliflower, coconut, cucumber, caterpillar**).

Try working with the same words until the child can say the words correctly in the games and activities most of the time, e.g. 70 per cent of the time. Then add some more words or change the set you are working on.

Try rotating sets of words. For example, work on up to ten words for a week and then work on a set of up to ten different words for another week, and another set of ten words for the third week; then go back to working on the first set of words.

Play games in small groups. This will increase the opportunities the child has to hear words with **k** and it will be fun!

Tell a story (Listening and speaking activity)

Aim
To say the words beginning and ending in the speech sound **k** in phrases and sentences in games and activities.

How?
By giving the child opportunities to hear, and see, you say words in phrases and sentences and to practise saying the words.

Resources
- At least five small pictures, e.g. **Kate, coal, kite, kiss, cork**.

- A computer or pen and paper to write a story, or a tape recorder or video recorder to record the child telling the story.

Instructions

1 Put the pictures face down in a pile in front of the child.

2 Turn over the first picture and make up the beginning of a story using the word, e.g. **Kate**. 'Once upon a time there was a very strong girl called Kate.'

3 Take it in turns to take a picture and make up the next part of the story using the word on it, e.g. **kite**.

'One day Kate was walking home from school when she met a boy crying. "Why are you crying?", she asked him.

"I've lost my new kite", he told her.'
Put the pictures face up on the table in a line as you use them in the story.

4 When you have finished the story, use the pictures to help the child remember and retell the story. Write the story on a computer or on paper or record it.

Make up sentences (Listening and speaking activity)

Aim

To say the words beginning and ending in the speech sound **k** in phrases and sentences in games and activities.

How?

By giving the child opportunities to hear, and see, you say words in phrases and sentences and to practise saying the words.

Resources

• At least six small pictures, e.g. **book**, **duck**, **sock**, **fork**, **lock**, **shark**.

• Paper and crayons, felt-tip pens or coloured pencils.

Instructions

1 Put the pictures face down in a pile in front of the child.

2 Take it in turns to take a picture, e.g. **sock**, put the word in a phrase, e.g. 'a smelly **sock**', or in a sentence, e.g. 'I've lost my **sock**!'

3 Take it in turns to turn over two pictures, e.g. **shark** and **book**, and put both words in a phrase, e.g. '**shark** in a **book**', or a sentence, e.g. 'I saw a **shark** reading a **book**!'

4   Increase the number of pictures so that you increase the number of words that you have to put into a phrase or sentence, e.g. 'I saw a **shark** reading a **book** to a **duck**, which was wearing **socks** and eating lunch with a **fork**.' See who can make the longest sentence!

5   See how many words the child can remember.

Variations

- Write the phrases or sentences and illustrate them. Cover up the writing so that the child can see the illustration only. See if she can remember the phrase or sentence.

- Choose at least four words and make up a short rhyme or poem using the words.

- Take it in turns to throw a dice to see how many words you have to use in a sentence, e.g. five, and make a sentence containing that many words, e.g. 'A **shark** read a book to a **duck**, which was eating lunch with a **fork** and wearing a **sock** on the **lake**.'

- See how many words that start or end with **k** the child can use in a sentence in one minute. Use a one-minute salt timer.

Make a word web (Listening and speaking activity)

Aim

To say the words beginning and ending in the speech sound **k** in phrases and sentences in games and activities.

How?

By giving the child opportunities to hear, and see, you say words in phrases and sentences and to practise saying the words.

Resources

- At least four small pictures, e.g. **cooker**, **camel**, **comic**, **cucumber**.

- Paper, or a work book, or a photocopy of the blank template for a word web. (p. 185)

- Pencils, crayons or felt-tip pens.

Instructions

1   Let the child choose one of the small pictures. Draw a circle in the middle of the piece of paper and write the word in it, e.g. **cucumber**. Ask the child to draw it so that you have a picture and the word.

2   Ask the child questions about the word. For example: 'What is a **cucumber**?'; e.g. food, a vegetable. 'Where does it live?'

   'Where do you find it?'; e.g. in shops, in the fridge, in salads. 'What does it look like?'; e.g. it is green and long.

   'What does it do?' 'What do you do with it?'; e.g. you eat it, you cut it, you wash it. 'Can you think of another vegetable?' 'Do you like cucumber?'

3   Make a word web by drawing lines radiating out from the circle containing the word the child has chosen. Write the child's answers at the end of each line you have drawn, or in a shape at the end of each line, e.g. square, circle, triangle, or along each line. For example: 1 It is a vegetable. 2 You find it in a shop (in a grocer's) 3 You can eat it.

4   Keep the word webs in a work book or a word bag or folder. When you have at least three word webs, choose one.

   Make sure the child cannot see it. Tell the child about the word and ask her to guess what it is, e.g. 'It's a vegetable. You find it in shops and it is long and green. What is it?'

5   Reverse this activity with older children so that they choose a picture and give you clues to guess what it is.

Board game variation (Speaking activity)

Aim
To say the words beginning and ending in the speech sound **k** in phrases and sentences in games and activities.

How?
By giving the child opportunities to hear, and see, you say words in phrases and sentences and to practise saying the words.

Resources
- A board game, e.g. snakes and ladders.

- A set of the adjective cards, e.g. *big*, *hot*, *shiny* (p. 180).

- At least six small pictures of words you have been working on.

- A set of the emotions cards, e.g. *Say it in a happy voice. Say it in a sad voice. Say it in an angry voice* (p. 181).

Instructions

1   Set up the board game. Put the adjectives and the small pictures face down in
    two piles.

2   Take it in turns to take a card from each pile before you have your go, e.g. *big*,
    kangaroo.

3   Make a sentence using the two words, e.g. 'I saw a *big* **kangaroo** in the zoo.' Then
    have your go.

Variations

*   Set up a board game and put a pile of the emotions cards and a pile of the small
    pictures face down. Before each go, players take an emotions card, e.g. *Say it in an angry
    voice*, and a small picture, e.g. **kitten**, and say the word in the manner of the emotion.

*   Put a pile of the emotions cards and a pile of the small pictures face down. Take it in
    turns to take a card from each pile, e.g. *Say it in a tired voice* and **cat**, and say the word
    in the manner of the emotion. The other player has to guess what the emotion is.

*   Put a pile of the emotions cards and a pile of the small pictures face down. Take it in
    turns to take a card from each pile, e.g. '*Say it in a sad voice*' and **duck**. Make a phrase
    or sentence using the word, e.g. 'Feed a **duck**', and say it in the emotion you have
    taken, e.g. in a sad voice. See if the other player can guess what the emotion is.

Continue the sentence (Listening and speaking activity)

Aim
To say the words beginning and ending in the speech sound **k** in phrases and sentences in
games and activities.

How?
By giving the child opportunities to hear, and see, you say words in phrases and
sentences and to practise saying the words.

Resources
*   At least four small pictures, e.g. **coat**, **cat**, **comb**, **corn**.

Instructions
1   Put the small pictures face down in a pile.

2   You start by saying 'I went to the market and I bought a …' and take a picture from
    the pile, e.g. **coat**.

3   The child says 'I went to the market and I bought a **coat** and a …' and then takes a
    picture from the pile, e.g. **cat**.

4. Keep going until a player cannot remember all the items they bought.

Variations

• Leave the pictures face up to help players remember what they bought.

• Change the place, e.g. 'I went to Jamaica and I saw …'; 'I went to the Moon and I took …'.

Say the missing word (Listening and speaking activity)

Aim

To say the words beginning and ending in the speech sound **k** in phrases and sentences in games and activities

How?

By giving the child opportunities to hear, and see, you say words in phrases and sentences and to practise saying the words.

Resources

• At least one of the jingles that use the words you have been working on, e.g. 'Nen nan nin. Put your **core** in the bin.'

Instructions

1. Read the jingle to the child at the end of a few sessions so that she knows it well.

2. Read the jingle, but leave out a word that contains the speech sound **k** in some lines of the jingle (the number of words you leave out will depend on the level of the child), e.g. 'Nen nan nin. Put your _____ (**core**) in the bin'. See if the child can remember the word and complete the sentence.

3. Gradually leave out more words in the jingle and see if the child can remember them, e.g. 'Nee noo nar. Put the _____ (**key**) in the _____ (**car**)'

Variations

• If the child cannot remember the words you have omitted from jingles, sound them out, e.g. **k – ee** (**key**).

• The child listens, puts the speech sounds together to make the word and says it: **key**.

• Older children might be able to read some of the jingles with you.

Think of a word (Speaking activity)

Aim

To say the words beginning and ending in the speech sound **k** in phrases and sentences in games and activities.

How?

By giving the child opportunities to hear, and see, you say words in phrases and sentences and to practise saying the words.

Resources

- Photocopy of the grid template *Can you think of ...? (p. 182)* and pencils or pens.

Instructions

1   Read the first question on the handout with the child: '*Can you think of an animal that begins with the sound k?*'

2   The child has to think of a word that begins with the sound **k**, e.g. **cat**, **camel**, **kitten**, **cow**. Write his answer on the handout and ask the second question: '*Can you think of a food that begins with the sound k?*' Let the child look at the small pictures to help him think of answers if he needs support.

3   If the child can answer all the questions, you could add further questions or the child could ask you further questions of his own!

Variation

- Make the activity into a competition. Players write their answers and do not show each other what they have written until the end.

Would you rather ...? (Listening and speaking activity)

Aim

To say the words beginning and ending in the speech sound **k** in phrases and sentences in games and activities.

How?

By giving the child opportunities to hear, and see, you say words in phrases and sentences and to practise saying the words.

Resources

- The *Would you rather ...?* sheet (p. 183). Cut it up and put the pieces in a pile face down.

Instructions

1. Take the first card from the pile. Read it out loud, e.g. *'Would you rather feed a shark or feed a duck?'*

2. When the child answers the question, e.g. 'Feed a **duck**', ask her 'Why?'

3. When the child has answered the questions, take another card and answer it.

4. Take it in turns to answer the *Would you rather ...?* questions.

Variations

• Make your own *Would you rather ...?* questions using words with **k** that you have worked on in this book.

• Older children might be able to read some of the *Would you rather ...?* questions.

• Carry out a survey with older children, e.g. ask teachers and children at least four of the *Would you rather ...?* questions and present the results.

I like / don't like ... (Listening and speaking activity)

Aim

To say the words beginning and ending in the speech sound **k** in phrases and sentences in games and activities.

How?

By giving the child opportunities to hear, and see, you say words in phrases and sentences and to practise saying the words.

Resources

• The large *I like* and *I don't like* resource and the *I like /don't like ...* sheet giving different activities (p.184). Cut the sheet of paper up into cards and put the cards in a pile face down.

Instructions

1 Take the first card from the pile. Read the first part out loud, e.g. *'feeding ducks'*.

2 Put the card on the 'I like' square or on the 'I don't like' square, depending on whether you like feeding ducks or not. For example: 'I like feeding ducks'.

3 Tell the child at least one thing about feeding ducks, e.g. 'I feed the ducks every time I go to the park.'

4 Take it in turns to take a card, tell each other if you like it or not and tell each other one thing about it (see the cards for suggestions).

Variation

• Make your own versions using words with **k** that you have worked on in this book.

Adjectives

hot	cold	dirty
wet	big	small
long	short	hungry
thirsty	round	red
heavy	tall	shiny

Emotions cards

Say it in a tired voice	Say it in a loud voice	Say it in a surprised voice	Say it in a low voice
Say it in a happy voice	Say it in a quiet voice	Say it in an excited voice	Say it in a high voice
Say it in a sad voice	Say it in an angry voice	Say it in a scared voice	Say it in a bored voice

Can you think of ...

an animal that begins with k?	
a colour that begins with k?	
a food that begins with k?	
a job that begins with k?	
a country that begins with k?	
a piece of clothing that begins with k?	
a sport that begins with k?	
a part of the body that begins with k?	
a name that begins with k?	

Would you rather ...

Would you rather feed a shark or feed a duck? Why?	Would you rather smell a sock or smell a duck? Why?
Would you rather ride a bike up a mountain or ride a bike across a desert? Why?	Would you rather read 20 books or wash 20 socks? Why?
Would you rather eat worms with a fork or feed a shark worms with a fork? Why?	Would you rather kiss a camel or kiss a kangaroo? Why?
Would you rather ride a cow to school or ride a camel to school? Why?	Would you rather your mum came to school in a baseball cap or in your coat? Why?
Would you rather dance with a cat or play the piano with a cat? Why?	Would you rather be kicked by a kitten or by a duck? Why?
Would you rather be lost in the dark or lost in a park? Why?	Would you rather eat a caterpillar or eat a cauliflower? Why?
Would you rather play football with a cowboy or play basketball with a kangaroo? Why?	Would you rather eat a carrot with ice cream or eat a carrot with custard? Why?

I like / I don't like

I like	I don't like
fast cars + tell me one thing, e.g. your dream car	eating apple cores + tell me one thing, e.g. your favourite fruit
flying a kite + tell me one thing, e.g. where you fly your kite	making cakes + tell me one thing, e.g. what kind of cake you can make
eating corn + tell me one thing, e.g. whether you like tinned corn or corn on the cob	sharks + tell me one thing, e.g. where sharks live
riding a bike + tell me one thing, e.g. what colour your bike is	feeding ducks + tell me one thing, e.g. where you feed the ducks
playing in the park + tell me one thing, e.g. what you like playing on in the park	reading comics + tell me one thing, e.g. what your favourite comic is
reading a book + tell me one thing, e.g. what your favourite book is	eating carrots + tell me one thing, e.g. what your favourite vegetable is
cowboys + tell me one thing, e.g. what cowboys do	kangaroos + tell me one thing, e.g. what your favourite animal is

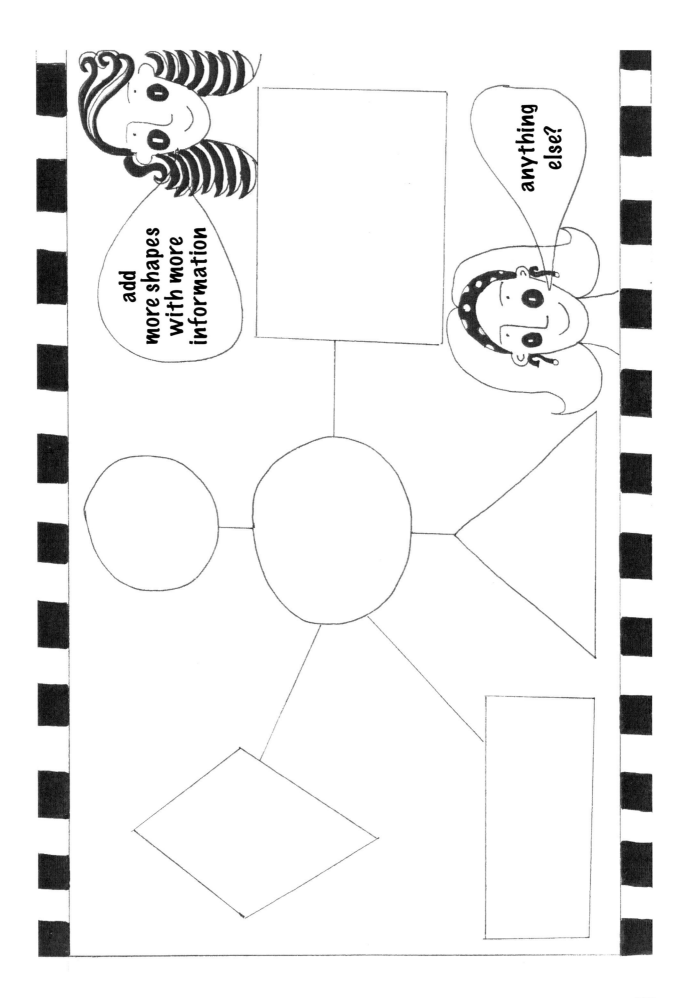

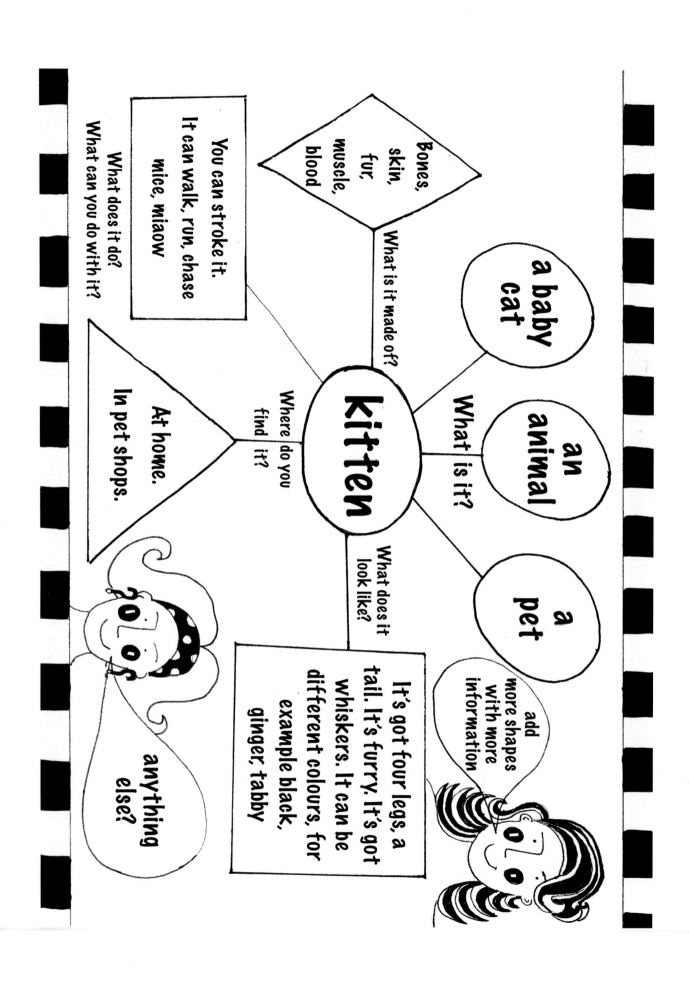

Kitten

a baby cat

an animal

a pet

What is it?

What is it made of?

Bones, skin, fur, muscle, blood

What can you do with it?
What does it do?

You can stroke it. It can walk, run, chase mice, miaow

Where do you find it?

At home. In pet shops.

What does it look like?

It's got four legs, a tail. It's furry. It's got whiskers. It can be different colours, for example black, ginger, tabby

add more shapes with more information

anything else?

SECTION 8

GAMES TO PLAY USING WORDS BEGINNING FROM ALL SECTIONS IN THE BOOK

Contents

Game 1: Pairs (Speaking game)

What you need to play

- At least two sets of small pictures of words you have been working on.

How to play

1 Shuffle the pictures and place them face down on the table.

2 Take it in turns to turn over two pictures.

3 Name each picture as you turn it over, e.g. '**Case**. **Cap**.'

4 If the pictures are the same, e.g. **cap** and **cap**, you keep the pair. If they are different, e.g. **case** and **cap**, you put them back on the table face down. The winner is the person who has the most pairs of pictures.

Game 2: Kim's game (Speaking game)

What you need to play

- At least one set of small pictures of words you have been working on.

How to play

1 Put at least three pictures in front of the child.

2 Name the pictures and talk about them with the child to make the pictures more memorable, e.g. '**Cap**. My son wears a **cap**. He has got a black and green **cap**.' '**Cat**. We've got a black and white **cat** like the one in the picture! He's a very fat **cat**!'

3 Tell the child to look at the pictures and 'take a photo' in his mind (mime taking a photo with an imaginary camera) to help him remember them.

4 Ask the child to close his eyes.

5 Take away one of the pictures.

6 Ask the child to open his eyes and see if he can remember what the missing picture is.

Variation

- Make the game more challenging by increasing the number of pictures you use and the number of pictures you take away when the child closes his eyes.

Game 3: Find the picture (Listening and speaking game)

What you need to play

- A set of small pictures of words you have been working on.

- Some Blu-Tack to stick the pictures around the room, e.g. on the door, on the back of a chair.

How to play

1 Show the child at least two pictures.

2 Name the pictures, e.g. 'Look! **Book** and **duck**'. Talk about them a little to help the child remember the pictures.

3 Ask the child to close her eyes.

4 Hide the pictures and ask the child to open her eyes.

5 Ask her to find one of the pictures, e.g. 'Find **book**.'

6 Reverse the game so that the child hides the pictures and tells you which one to find.

Variation

Make the game more challenging by increasing the number of pictures you hide and the number of pictures you ask the child to find. For example, hide four pictures and ask the child to find two of them.

Game 4: Find the coin (Listening and speaking game)

What you need to play

- A set of at least six small pictures of words you have been working on.

- A coin

How to play

1 Put at least six of the small pictures in front of the child.

2 Name the pictures with the child, e.g. '**Kite. Cake. Cot. Cap.**'

3 Tell the child to close his eyes.

4 Hide a coin under one of the pictures.

5   Tell the child to open his eyes. The aim of the game is to find the coin. The child has to say which picture he thinks the coin is under, e.g. **cot**. Keep a record of how many guesses the child has before he finds the coin.

6   Reverse the game so that the child hides the coin and you guess which picture it is under. The winner is the person who finds the coin with the least number of guesses.

Variation

Make the game more challenging by increasing the number of coins you hide. For example, hide three coins and the child has to guess which pictures they are under.

Game 5: Which picture? (Listening and speaking game)

What you need to play

*   A set of small pictures of words you have been working on.

*   Two cups (make sure you can't see through them).

*   A coin or a counter or a small toy that will fit under the cups.

How to play

1   Choose two pictures and name them with the child, e.g. '**Cow. Key.**'

2   Turn the cups upside-down and place them at the top of the pictures.

3   Tell the child to close her eyes and put the coin, counter or small toy under one of the cups.

4   Ask the child to open her eyes. The aim of the game is for the child to guess which cup the coin, counter or small toy is under. The child names the picture that the cup is on, e.g. '**cow**', and then looks under the cup to see if the item is underneath.

5   Reverse the game so that the child hides the item and you guess which cup it is under.

Game 6: Catch a picture (Listening and speaking game)

What you need to play

*   A set of small pictures of words you have been working on.

*   Paper clips to attach to the pictures that you are using in the game.

- A fishing rod. Make one by attaching some string to a piece of wood or a pencil and tie a small magnet to the end of the string.

How to play

1 Put a paper clip on each of the small pictures that you are using in the game. Place the pictures face down, so that you can't see the pictures, on a flat surface or in a large bowl or similar container.

2 Take turns to 'catch a fish' with the rod and name the picture, e.g. **camel**.

Variations

- See if you can catch a pair of pictures, e.g. **kitten** and **kitten**.

- Spread the pictures out picture side up and take it in turns to tell each other which picture to catch: e.g. 'Catch **kettle**,' 'Catch **kitchen** and **carpet**!' Make this game more challenging by increasing the number of pictures you ask each other to catch.

Game 7: Bowling (Listening and speaking game)

What you need to play

- Two plastic bottles or skittles

- A set of small pictures of words you have been working on.

- Blu-Tack to stick the pictures onto the bottles or skittles.

- A small ball

How to play

1 Choose two pictures of words you have been working on, e.g. **back** and **shark**.

2 Attach the pictures onto bottles or skittles with Blu-Tack, e.g. put **back** on one skittle and put **shark** on the other skittle, or put a picture under each skittle.

3 To play this game as a listening game, give the ball to the child. Name one of the pictures on one of the skittles, e.g. **shark**. The child listens and points to the picture that she heard you name. If she is right, she tries to knock over the skittle with the ball.

4 To play this game as a speaking game, let the child name one of the pictures, e.g. **back**. You listen and point to the picture that you heard her name. If you are right, you roll the ball and try to knock over the skittle.

Game 8: Goal! (Listening and speaking game)

What you need to play

- A set of small pictures of words you have been working on.

- A bean bag or a small ball

- Two boxes or containers, e.g. buckets

- Blu-Tack to stick the pictures onto the boxes or containers.

How to play

1   Choose two pictures of words that you have been working on, e.g. **car** and **core**. Attach the pictures to the containers or place them in front of the containers.

2   To play this game as a listening game, give the bean bag or ball to the child. Name one of the pictures, e.g. **car**. The child listens and points to the picture that he heard you name, i.e. car. If he is right, he tries to throw the bean bag or ball into the appropriate container.

3   To play this game as a speaking game, let the child name one of the pictures, e.g. **core**. You listen and point to the picture that you heard him name. If you are right, you throw the ball into the corresponding container.

Game 9: What is it? (Speaking game)

What you need to play

- At least one set of small pictures of words you have been working on.

- Plasticine or playdough

How to play

1   Put the pictures face down in a pile in front of the players.

2   Take a picture from the pile. Do not show it to anyone else.

3   Take some playdough or plasticine and make a model of the picture.

4   The child has to guess what it is.

5   Take it in turns to take a picture and make a model of it for the other player to guess what it is.

Variations

- Limit the number of guesses to three!

- Give the child a minute to guess what your model is! Use a one-minute salt timer.

Game 10: Draw a picture! (Speaking game)

What you need to play

- At least one set of small pictures of words you have been working on.

- Paper and pencils or pens

How to play

1 Put the pictures in a pile face down in front of the players.

2 Take a picture. Do not show it to anyone else.

3 Draw the picture.

4 Ask the child to guess what the picture is as you are drawing it.

5. Take it in turns to take a picture and draw it for the other player to guess what it is.

Variations

- Limit the number of guesses to six or fewer!

- Give the child a minute to guess what your picture is! Use a one-minute salt timer.

Game 11: Guess what? (Listening and speaking game)

What you need to play

- At least one set of small pictures of words you have been working on.

How to play

1 Choose a picture. Do not show it to anyone else.

2 Describe the picture for the child to guess what it is, e.g. 'Babies sleep in it. It is made of wood and it has high sides so that the baby can't get out.' (**cot**)

3   If this is too difficult for the child, put at least three pictures in front of the child and describe one of them. The child listens to your description and points to the picture.

4   Reverse the game where possible so that the child describes the picture and you guess what it is.

Variations

• Limit the number of clues you give the child to four or fewer!

• Give the child a minute to guess what your picture is! Use a one-minute salt timer.

Game 12: Listen and colour (Listening and speaking game)

What you need to play

• Two identical sets of small pictures of words you have been working on; one for you and one for the child. Do not laminate them.

• A barrier which you can place between yourself and the child so that you cannot see each other's pictures.

How to play

1   With younger children, e.g. aged three to four, put at least two pictures in front of the child, e.g. **camel** and **cooker**.

2   Ask the child to colour one of the pictures, e.g. 'Colour the **cooker**.' To make the game more challenging increase the number of pictures and the number of colours. For example: 'Colour the **camel** red and the **cooker** green.' 'Colour the **camel's** legs blue and his nose orange.'

3   With children over four, make this game more challenging by placing a barrier between yourself and the child so that you cannot see each other's pictures. Put at least two pictures behind the barrier. Colour one of the pictures, or colour both of them using different colours. Then give instructions to the child, e.g. 'Colour the **camel** green and the **cooker** blue.' When the child has finished, remove the barrier to see if you have coloured the same pictures.

4   Reverse the game where possible so that the child gives you instructions.

Game 13: Listen and do (Listening and speaking game)

What you need to play

- Two identical sets of small pictures of words you have been working on; one for you and one for the child.

- A selection of objects that are small enough to put on the pictures, e.g. a toy car, a button, a teaspoon, a toy animal, a small teddy bear. You need two of each so that you and the child have the same objects to play this game.

- A barrier that you can place between yourself and the child so that you cannot see each other's pictures.

How to play

1 Choose at least two pictures, e.g. **cow** and **key**, and two objects, e.g. a toy pig and a button. Put the objects on the pictures on your side of the barrier so that the child cannot see them. For example, put the pig on the picture of the **key** and the button on the picture of the **cow**.

2 Ask the child to do the same, e.g. 'Put the pig on the **key** and the button on the **car**'.

3 When he has finished, raise the barrier to see if he has the same pictures and objects as you.

4 Reverse the game so that the child gives the instructions and you listen and do.

Game 14: Charades (Speaking game)

What you need to play

- A set of actions to perform, e.g. *Stroke a cat!* (p. 197)

How to play

1 Put the actions in a pile face down.

2 Take it in turns to pick up an action and mime what it says, e.g. *Ride a camel!*

3 The winner is the person who guesses the most mimes correctly.

Variations

- Make up mimes with the child using the words you have been working on.

Charades

Stroke a cat!	Open the door with a key!
Eat an apple and put the core in the bin!	Play in the park!
Milk a cow!	Fly a kite!
Feed a duck!	Cut someone's hair!
Ride a bike!	Read a book!
Comb your hair!	Smell a smelly sock!
Ride a camel!	Swim in the lake!
Jump like a kangaroo!	Put the shopping in the cupboard!
Give a carrot to a rabbit!	Light a candle and blow it out!
Be a cowboy!	Pick up a caterpillar and hold it on your hand!

SECTION 9

SESSION PLANS

Section 9: **Session plans**

Session plans for a child aged three and a half to seven years old, who is not saying the speech sound **k** in his talking. He may say **t** instead of **k**, e.g. **tar** instead of **car**, **tea** instead of **key**, or he may say **g** instead of **k**, e.g. **goat** instead of **coat**.

Aim

To help the child say the speech sound **k** in his talking.

How?

• By showing him how his mouth works, e.g. tongue movements, lip movements.

• By helping him to hear the speech sound **k** and the speech sound **k** at the beginning and end of words. The child might think he is saying **k**, so he thinks others can understand what he wants to tell them. You need to help him realise that he is not saying **k**, which can make it hard for others to understand what he wants to say.

• By helping him to make the speech sound **k** and then say **k** in words, e.g. **key**, **can**, **book**.

1 To help the child to say the speech sound k – Section 1 and Section 2.

What?	Why?	How?	Next step?
Mouth exercises	To help the child learn about his mouth and movements we make for speech.	**Section 1** 1. Look in a mirror, e.g. 'Show me your tongue. Show me your teeth.' 2. Do single movements together with a mirror, e.g. 'Can you put your tongue up to your nose?'	**This is easy:** Sequence movements in Section 1, e.g. *Can you move your tongue up to your nose and then down to your chin?* Play suggested games in Section 1 to practise sequences of mouth movements, e.g. roll dice to get a number and do mouth movements that number of times. **This is hard:** Keep working on single movements using a mirror.
Listening games	To help the child hear the speech sound **k**. To help the child hear that **t** and **k** are different speech sounds.	**Section 2** 1. Do the listening activities in Section 2, e.g. 'Listen, when you hear me say **k**, put a cat on a cushion.' 2. Play the listening games from Section 8, e.g. *Bowling* (stick **k** on one skittle and another speech sound on the other; see the list of speech sounds and the ages most children start to say them on p. 1), *Catch a picture, Listen and colour.* 3. Play a listening game with the drawing activity in Section 2, e.g. 'When I say **k**, colour in a ring.'	**This is easy:** Play the variation of this listening activity in Section 1 (listen to more speech sounds and put a cat on a cushion when you hear **k**, e.g. **m, s, p, w, k**). Use more than two speech sounds in activities, e.g. put **k, p, t** on skittles. Make sure the speech sounds you use in games are very different to make it easier for the child to hear **k**, e.g. **w, k, b, s**. **This is hard:** Play the listening games with a toy or a puppet so that the child can watch and listen.

201

What?	Why?	How?	Next step?
Speaking games	To help the child say the speech sound **k**.	**Section 2** 1. Use a mirror so that the child can see your mouth and his mouth. Put a **cat** on a **cushion** or a **crown** on a **king** or a **candle** on a **cake** and say **k**. Take turns to say **k** in this activity. 2. Use the drawing activities in Section 2 to practise saying **k**, e.g. 'Say **k** and draw an eye on the alien.' 3. Use **k** and other speech sounds in the speaking games in Section 8, e.g. *Kim's game* (present at least three speech sounds, e.g. **k, s, b,** the child closes his eyes and you take away one), *Pairs, Which picture?*	**This is easy:** Start working on words that begin with **k** in Section 3 (**key, car, cow, core, Kay, Kai**). **This is hard:** 1. See tips on helping children to say **k**. 2. Do mouth movements to help child learn about his mouth. 3. Play listening games so the child has lots of opportunities to hear **k** but does not feel any pressure to try to say **k**.

2 To help the child say k at the beginning of short words – Section 1 and Section 3

What?	Why?	How?	Next step?
Mouth exercises	To help the child learn about his mouth and movements we make for speech.	**Section 1** 1. Look in a mirror, e.g. 'Show me your tongue. Show me your teeth.' 2. Do single movements together with a mirror, e.g. '*Can you put your tongue up to your nose and then down to your chin?*.'	**This is easy:** Sequence movements in Section 1, e.g. 'Can you move your tongue side to side?' Play suggested games in Section 1 to practise sequences of mouth movements, e.g. roll dice to get a number and do mouth movements that number of times, e.g. four. **This is hard:** Keep working on single movements using a mirror.
Listening games	To help the child hear the speech sound **k** in words.	**Section 3** 1. Do the listening activities in Section 3, e.g. present at least two pictures to the child, name one of them and the child holds up the one he heard you say. With children over four and a half years old, play the listening games where you sound words out for the child, e.g. **c – ow (cow)**. 2. Play the listening games from the list of games in Section 8 using the words in Section 3, e.g. *Bowling, Catch a picture, Listen and colour*. 3. Read the jingles from Section 3 to the child.	**This is easy:** Play the listening games from Section 4. Play the listening games with words that rhyme with the **k** words you are using, but start with **t**, e.g. **car** and **tar**, **Kai** and **tie**, **core** and **tore**, **key** and **tea**. For example, play *Catch a picture, Listen and colour*. **This is hard:** Play the listening games with a toy or a puppet so that the child can watch and listen. Go back to playing listening games with **k**, and with **k** and other speech sounds, so that the child has more opportunities to hear the sounds before you work on **k** in words.

What?	Why?	How?	Next step?
Speaking games	To help the child say the speech sound **k** in words.	**Section 3** 1. Play the speaking games from Section 3, e.g. What's the picture, Hide the cat, Roll the dice for a shape and number. 2. Play the speaking games in Section 8 using the words from Section 3. 3. See tips at the end of Section 3 on using jingles as speaking activities, e.g. leaving a word out of a line of a jingle for the child to say.	**This is easy:** Start working on words that begin with **k** in Section 4, e.g. **comb, corn, can, coat, cat.** **This is hard:** See the tips in Section 3 for help. Go back to working on Section 2 and gradually introduce words and games from Section 3.

3 To help the child say k at the beginning of longer words – Section 1 and Section 4.

Tip: Some children find it easier to say k at the end of words than at the beginning. If the child you are working with finds it easier to say k at the end of words, work on words from Section 5 before you work on words from Section 4.

What?	Why?	How?	Next step?
Mouth exercises	To help the child learn about his mouth and movements we make for speech. To warm up before starting work on saying **k** in words.	**Section 1** Sequence mouth movements. Play mouth movement games from Section 1.	**This is easy:** Tell the child you are warming up before the hard work begins like footballers and athletes do before a game or a race! Keep this section short and fun. **This is hard:** Keep working on single movements using a mirror.
Listening games	To help the child hear the speech sound **k** in words.	**Section 4** 1. Do the listening activities in Section 4, e.g. *Listen and guess, What did I say?* With children over four and a half years old, play the listening games where you sound out words for the child, e.g. **c – ow** (**cow**). 2. Play the listening games in Section 8 using the words in Section 4, e.g. *Goal!*	**This is easy:** Play the listening games from Section 5. **This is hard:** Play the listening games with a toy or a puppet so that the child can watch and listen. Go back to Section 3.

What?	Why?	How?	Next step?
Speaking games	To help the child say the speech sound **k** in words.	**Section 4** 1. Play speaking games from Section 4, e.g. *Roll the dice, Say the word.* 2. Play the speaking games in Section 8 using the words from Section 4, e.g. *Guess what?* 3. See the tips on using jingles as speaking activities, e.g. leaving a word out of a line of a jingle for the child to say.	**This is easy:** Start working on words that end with **k** in Section 5, e.g. **book, duck, sock.** **This is hard:** See the tips in Section 4 for help. Go back to working on Section 3 and gradually introduce words and games from Section 4.

4 To help the child say k at the end of words – Section 1 and Section 5

What?	Why?	How?	Next step?
Mouth exercises	To help the child learn about his mouth and movements we make for speech. To warm up before starting work on saying **k** in words.	**Section 1** Sequence mouth movements. Play mouth movement games from Section 1.	**This is easy:** Tell the child you are warming up before the hard work begins like footballers and athletes do before a game or a race! Keep this section short and fun. **This is hard:** Keep working on single movements using a mirror.
Listening games	To help the child hear **k** in words.	**Section 5** 1. Do the listening activities in Section 5, e.g. *Listen and guess, What did I say?* With children over four and a half years of age, play the listening games where you sound words out for the child, e.g. **boo – k.** 2. Play the listening games from the list of games in Section 8, e.g. *What is it? Catch a picture*, using the words in Section 5. 3. Read the jingles from Section 5 to the child. See the tips on reading the jingles at the end of Section 3.	**This is easy:** Play the listening games from Section 6. Use the words from Section 5 and play the listening games from earlier sections. **This is hard:** Play the listening games with a toy or a puppet so that the child can watch and listen. Go back to working on Section 4 and gradually introduce words from Section 5.

207

What?	Why?	How?	Next step?
Speaking games	To help the child say the speech sound **k** in words.	**Section 5** 1. Play speaking games from Section 5, e.g. *Roll the dice, What's the word?* 2. Play the speaking games in Section 8, e.g. Kim's game, using the words from Section 5. 3. See the tips on using jingles as speaking activities at the end of Section 3, e.g. leaving a word out of a line of a jingle for the child to say.	**This is easy:** Start working on Section 6. **This is hard:** See the tips in Section 5 for help. Go back to working on Section 4 and gradually introduce words and games from Section 5.

5 To help the child say k in words with more than one syllable – Section 1 and Section 6 (games from other sections using words from Section 6 optional)

What?	Why?	How?	Next Step?
Mouth exercises	To help the child learn about his mouth and movements we make for speech. To warm up before starting work on saying **k** in words.	**Section 1** Sequence mouth movements. Play mouth movement games from Section 1.	**This is easy:** Tell the child you are warming up before the hard work begins like footballers and athletes do before a game or a race! Keep this section short and fun. **This is hard:** Keep working on single movements using a mirror.
Listening games	To help the child hear **k** in words.	**Section 6** 1. Listening activities in Section 6, e.g. *What did I say?* 2. Play the listening games in Section 8 using the words in Section 6.	**This is easy:** Great! The child can hear the speech sound **k** at the beginning and end of words. **This is hard:** Play the listening games with a toy or a puppet so that the child can watch and listen. Go back to Section 5 and gradually introduce words from Section 6.

209

What?	Why?	How?	Next step?
Speaking games	To help the child say the speech sound **k** in words.	**Section 6** 1. Play the speaking games from Section 6, e.g. *Finish my word*. 2. Play the speaking games in Section 8 using the words from Section 6. 3. See the tips on using jingles as speaking activities at the end of Section 3, e.g. leaving a word out of a line of a jingle for the child to say.	**This is easy:** Start working using words from the sections you have covered in phrases or sentences in Section 7. **This is hard:** See the tips in Section 6 for help. Go back to working on Sections 5 and 4 and gradually introduce words and games from Section 6.

6 To help the child say k in words in phrases and sentences – Section 7

What?	Why?	How?	Next step?
Using words that the child has worked on in the book in phrases and sentences in games and activities	To help the child say the speech sound **k** in their talking.	See the tips in Section 7 for using activities, e.g. how to choose words to work on. Play games little and often, e.g. play a game from Section 7 at least three times a week.	**This is easy:** Play games in groups, not just one-to-one with the child. Give activities to carers to play at home. **This is hard:** Play games one-to-one, keep playing games that are familiar to the child from the list of games in Section 8.

211

What next?
- Make lists of words that contain **k**. Choose words that are useful for the child, for example names of family, friends, teachers, classmates, pets, towns, cities, television programmes, food. If you are working in a nursery or school, use topic or curriculum vocabulary if you can so that the child has more opportunities to hear these words and try to use them. For example, if the topic is our environment, the words could be: market, café, tennis courts, cottage, etc.

- Use five to ten words, depending on the child. Ask older children if there are any words that have **k** in them that they find difficult to say and would like to work on.

- Make a list of the words and then make at least two copies of the words (so that you can play games like *Pairs*), and cut them into word cards. Make a word box or word bag to keep the words in. Try to work on words at least twice a week for at least ten minutes each time. Follow the same procedure in each session.

Suggested sessions
- Take it in turns to take a word out of the bag or box. Say each word for the child, so that she can hear the word.

- Ask the child to say the word after you. Aim for the best production she can do. Help her if she finds it hard by breaking words into chunks (see the tips on saying longer words and on saying **k** at the end of words for advice and examples). Try breaking words into syllables, e.g. **cal – en – dar**. Try starting at the end of the word, e.g. **der – lender – calendar**. Keep this activity short.

Tips
- Ask the child to imagine saying the word before she tries to say it out loud.

- Ask the child to say the word to herself quietly at least three times and then say it out loud to you.

- Put a rhythm on longer words, e.g. tap them with your finger or nod your head as you say them, or do bigger movements, e.g. bend your knees on each syllable.

- Choose one or two activities or games from this book to practise saying words.

- When the child can say her words accurately at least 70 per cent of the time, add some more words. Keep a checklist of the words so that you can see progress.

- Review words regularly by taking a few out of the word bag or box and playing games and activities with them from this book.

- When the child is making good progress with the words, give her opportunities to use them in the nursery or classroom, e.g. using names that contain **k**, talking about the topic that the words are from.

References

Flynn L & Lancaster G (1996) *Children's Phonology Sourcebook*, Speechmark Publishing, Milton Keynes.

Grunwell P (1987) *Clinical Phonology*, 2nd edn, Croom Helm, London.

Holm A, Crosbie S & Dodd B (2005) 'Phonological approaches to intervention', in Dodd B (ed), *Differential Diagnosis and Treatment of Children with Speech Disorder* (2nd edn), Whurr Publishers, London.

Ripley K, Daines B & Barrett J (1997) *Dyspraxia: a Guide for Teachers and Parents,* David Fulton Publishers, London.

Stackhouse J (1992) 'Promoting reading and spelling skills through speech therapy', Fletcher P & Hall D (eds) *Specific Speech and Language Disorders in Children*, Whurr Publishers, London.